A Practical Guide to
Health Assessment

A Practical Guide to
Health Assessment
second edition

Marilyn Shelley Leasia, RN, MSN, FNP

Nurse Practitioner
Department of Medicine
Montefiore Medical Center
Bronx, New York

Frances Donovan Monahan, PhD, RN

Professor and Coordinator
Department of Nursing
SUNY Rockland Community College
Suffern, New York

W. B. SAUNDERS COMPANY
An imprint of Elsevier Science

W. B. SAUNDERS COMPANY
An imprint of Elsevier Science

The Curtis Center
Independence Square West
Philadelphia, Pennsylvania 19106

Library of Congress Cataloging-in-Publication Data

Leasia, Marilyn Shelley.
    A practical guide to health assessment / Marilyn Shelley Leasia,
Frances Donovan Monahan.—2nd ed.
        p. cm.
    ISBN 0–7216–8989–2
    1. Nursing assessment. I. Monahan, Frances Donovan. II. Title.
RT48 .L43 2002
616.07′5—dc21

                                                                    2001049411

Vice President, Publishing Director, Nursing: Sally Schrefer
Executive Editor: Robin Carter
Associate Developmental Editor: Barbara Cicalese
Production Manager: Donna L. Morrissey

A PRACTICAL GUIDE TO HEALTH ASSESSMENT

ISBN 0721689892

Printed in the United States of America

Last digit is the print number: 9   8   7   6   5   4   3   2   1

*Dedicated with love
to my husband Isdor Sobze
and our wonderful daughters
Dora, Pamela, and Jessica.*

MARILYN SHELLEY LEASIA

*Dedicated to the memory of
my husband William T. Monahan,
my son Michael McCain Monahan,
my daughter Kerryane Torpey Monahan,
and my aunt Claire T. Torpey.*

FRANCES D. MONAHAN

Preface

The rapidly changing health care delivery system has made strong history-taking, physical examination skills essential for today's practitioners. However, until now, only large textbooks provided the detailed, heavily illustrated content necessary to learning health assessment.

Our aim with this book is to provide students with a portable guide that is easy to use and provides the detailed information they need to take a client's health history and perform a physical examination. The content is presented in clear, step-by-step increments, with the liberal use of illustrations to help reinforce learning.

Using a body systems approach, each chapter addresses the entire life span by including both pediatric (see [ABC] icon) and geriatric (see icon) considerations. We have included transcultural content to address the needs of our diverse client population. Transcultural content is indicated by the icon and blue italicized type within the chapters.

In this edition, we have also added Focused Rapid Assessment boxes to guide learners in assessment of patients presenting with selected common symptoms. Also, we've added an Appendix about Pain, the fifth vital sign.

By combining our respective areas of expertise as nurse practitioner and educator, we have worked to reconcile the reality of clinical practice with the needs of today's students. We think you will agree the result is a book that will not only teach the skills of history taking and physical examination but will leave the reader with a true understanding of the importance of health assessment.

MARILYN SHELLEY LEASIA
FRANCES D. MONAHAN

Acknowledgments

The authors wish to thank Robin Carter, Executive Editor; Barbara Cicalese, Associate Developmental Editor; and Pat Morrison, Art and Design Director of W. B. Saunders Company.

A special thank you to Sue Anne Eitches, Ellen Flynn, Janet Drew Reynolds, and Joan Stackhouse, contributors to the first edition of this text, whose excellent work helped make this edition possible.

Contents

The Health History

The health history is a collection of subjective data that includes information on both the patient's past and present health status. It is used in conjunction with the physical examination and laboratory findings as a basis for drawing conclusions about an individual's state of health. It allows positive aspects of health and health habits as well as abnormal symptoms, health problems, health teaching needs, and health concerns to be identified.

COMPONENTS OF A COMPREHENSIVE HEALTH HISTORY

Date history obtained

Source of history (patient, spouse, relative, friend, medical records, etc.)

Interpreter if used (name, role, or relationship to patient)

Reason for seeking health care (e.g., routine physical examination, referral by another health care provider, presence of signs or symptoms of illness); record in patient's own words

Patient Profile Data

Name

Address

Telephone number

Social Security number

Date of birth (day, month, year)

Place of birth (city, state, country)

Sex

Race/ethnic origin

Marital status (single, married, divorced, widowed)

Religious preference (religion as well as name of house of worship, spiritual advisor if appropriate)

Education

Occupation

Hobbies

Military service

Name of physician

Source of referral

Insurance information (Medicare/Medicaid number, other insurance name and number)

Present Illness Data

Date of onset

Symptoms (type, location, frequency, duration)

Precipitating and/or associated factors

Relieving and alleviating factors (e.g., timing, setting)

Effect on other body functions

Effect on ADLs and life-style

Treatment measures utilized (type and frequency)

Effectiveness of treatment measures

Present Health Status (Apart from Present Illness)

Perceived state of health apart from current illness (patient's perception of self as healthy, prone to specific ailments, always having some health problem, etc.)

Existing health problems apart from the present illness (type, management)

Physical handicaps (type, management)

Prescription medications currently taken (name, dose, route, frequency, for how long, by whom prescribed, reason for taking, side effects)

OTC medications including herbal remedies and dietary supplements (name, dose, frequency, reason for taking, effectiveness)

(Also question regarding use of borrowed drugs. Be sure to warn of the dangers of this practice after asking; do not warn prior to asking as it could make the patient hesitant to admit to their use.)

Home remedies used (type, frequency, reason for use, effectiveness)

Complementary/alternative therapies used

Allergies (food, drug, environmental; type of reaction, management)

Immunization status (dates and types, e.g., measles/mumps/rubella, polio, pertussis/tetanus, tetanus booster, influenza, diphtheria, hepatitis; pneumococcal pneumonia) (see Appendix 1)

Past Personal Health Data

Childhood illnesses (e.g., strep throat, scarlet fever, rheumatic fever, polio, measles, mumps, rubella, chicken pox)

Serious adult illnesses (e.g., diabetes, hypertension, heart disease, cancer; treatment)

Accidents/injuries (type, date, treatment, sequelae)

Hospitalizations (date, cause, hospital, physician, treatment, length of stay)

Surgery (date, type, postoperative course, name of hospital and surgeon)

Obstetric history (number of pregnancies, viable deliveries; course of completed pregnancies, type of labor and delivery; sex, weight, and general condition of each neonate; postpartum course; number of spontaneous abortions, number of therapeutic abortions, age of pregnancy at time of each abortion)

Exposure to toxins or environmental pollutants (type, amount of exposure, untoward effects)

Blood transfusions (dates, number, untoward effects)

Family Medical Data

Age and health, or age and cause of death of parents, grandparents, siblings

Blood relative history of heart disease, hypertension, cerebrovascular disease, diabetes, anemia, cancer, arthritis, alcoholism, obesity, tuberculosis, renal disorders, seizure disorders, or mental illness (specific disease, age of onset, management)

Communicable disease in close family members, including spouse and children (type, date of onset, treatment)

Age and health history of spouse and children

Record family history in diagram or genogram form for easy reference (Fig. 1–1).

Life-Style Data

Ability to perform basic ADLs, such as:

- toileting
- bathing
- grooming
- dressing
- walking
- climbing stairs
- eating
- using the telephone
- shopping
- cooking
- housekeeping/cleaning
- laundry
- managing money
- transportation
- taking medications

(Indicate ability as I—*independent;* A—*needs assistance;* D—*dependent.*)

Usual daily activities

Work (type, responsibilities, hours, attitude toward, stresses/ problems)

Perceived role in family unit

Exercise patterns (type, frequency, duration)

Leisure activities/hobbies (type, time involved)

Participation in social groups (type, amount)

Sexual orientation

Sexual activity (frequency, type, use of contraceptives)

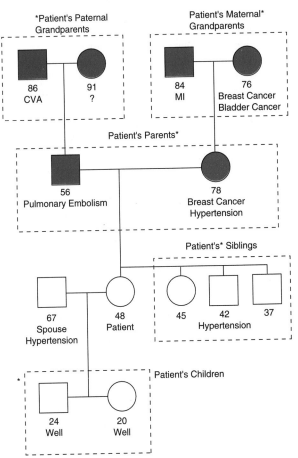

FIGURE 1-1 Family medical history recorded as a genogram.

Rest/sleep (usual sleep time; quality of sleep; difficulty falling alseep, staying asleep, or waking up; sleep aids used; sleep routine (e.g., light on, music))

Nutritional intake (time, type and amount of foods and fluids typically consumed in a 24-hour period, recent change in appetite, special diet)

Eating habits

Adequate finances for food

Caffeine intake (source, amount, pattern of use)

Use of alcohol (type, pattern of use, amount used, number of years used, effect of use on work and other activities)

Use of tobacco (type, amount per day, number of years used)

Use of "stop smoking" products such as nicotine patches, nicotine gums, etc

Use of illegal drugs (type, pattern of use, amount used, number of years used)

Recent trips to foreign countries (specify)

Health Management Data

Understanding of personal health status

Personal health goals

Routine hygienic practices (type, frequency, cultural taboos)

Date of last physical examination

Health screening tests (e.g., mammogram, Pap smear, stool for occult blood; type, date, results)

Self-examination (e.g., breast, testicular, skin; date of most recent self-examination; frequency; technique)

Date of most recent dental examination

Date of most recent eye examination

Date of most recent hearing examination

Date and results of most recent PPD or chest x-ray

Date and result of most recent ECG

Expectations of health care workers

Psychosocial Data

Perception of self (e.g., strengths, weaknesses, appearance, ability to function)

Sources of personal stress

Ability to cope (coping mechanisms used in the past, methods of relieving stress, persons/things that aid coping)

Perceived effect of feelings about present illness

Significant others (who, relationship to patient, location)

Family relationships (family members, proximity of residence, type of interaction between and among family members, patient's role in the family, how and by whom family decisions are made, how family copes with problems, how family is coping with the patient's illness)

Religious practices desired during illness (e.g., bible reading; visit from minister, hospital chaplain, medicine man, faith healer; wearing of medals; wearing of a medicine bag)

Home environment

- Type (e.g., house or apartment, number of rooms, owned or rented, one or more stories, number of stairs)
- Facilities in home (e.g., telephone, heat, furnishings in good repair)
- Number and age of others in household
- Type of neighborhood (e.g., urban, suburban, or rural; traffic; sidewalks; gangs; amount of crime)
- Available transportation (car, bus, walking)
- Access to shopping, house of worship, drug store, health care facilities, education facilities
- Type of (elderly, or mix of ages, none during the day, working) and relationship to neighbors

History of physical or sexual abuse (dates, type, by whom, action taken, stage of problem resolution)

Recent changes in life style

 Support system available (note cultural variations (life ways) that affect support, such as Mexican-American succorama)

Review of Systems

See history and current status questions at beginning of Chapters 3 through 22. Remember, when obtaining a history of signs and symptoms, explore all the areas identified in the PQRST mnemonic as shown in Table 1–1.

GUIDELINES FOR OBTAINING A HEALTH HISTORY

Greet patient by name using appropriate title (e.g., Mr., Mrs., Ms., Reverend, Sister, Doctor).

Introduce yourself, giving your name, title, and role.

Provide a private, quiet environment free of interruptions.

TABLE 1-1	The PQRST Mnemonic: System of Evaluation of Symptoms			
Provocative or Palliative	Quality or Quantity	Region or Radiation	Severity Scale	Timing
What causes the symptom? What makes it better or worse? ■ First occurrence. What were you doing when you first experienced or noticed the symptom? What seems to trigger it: stress? position? certain activities? arguments? (For a physical symptom such as a discharge: What seems to cause it or make it worse? For a psychological symptom: Does the depression occur when you feel	**How does the symptom feel, look, or sound? How much of it are you experiencing now?** ■ Quality. How would you describe the symptom—how it feels, looks, or sounds? ■ Quantity. How much are you experiencing now? Is it so much that it prevents you from performing any activities? Is it more or less than you experienced at any other time?	**Where is the symptom located? Does it spread?** ■ Region. Where does the symptom occur? ■ Radiation. In the case of pain, does it travel down your back or arms, up your neck, or down your legs?	**How does the symptom rate on a severity scale of 1 to 10, with 10 being the most extreme?** ■ Severity. How bad is the symptom at its worst? Does it force you to lie down, sit down, or slow down? ■ Course. Does the symptom seem to be getting better, getting worse, or staying about the same?	**When did the symptom begin? How often does it occur? Is it sudden or gradual?** ■ Onset. On what date did the symptom first occur? What time did it begin? ■ Type of onset. How did the symptom start: suddenly? gradually? ■ Frequency. How often do you experience the symptom: hourly? daily? weekly? monthly? When do you usually experience it: during the day? at night? in the early

rejected?) What relieves the symptom: changing diet? changing position? taking medication? being active?
■ Aggravation. What makes the symptom worse?

morning? Does it awaken you? Does it occur before, during, or after meals? Does it occur seasonally?
■ Duration. How long does an episode of the symptom last?

From Morton PG. Health Assessment in Nursing. 2nd ed. Philadelphia: FA Davis, 1993.

Ensure that the patient is as comfortable as possible prior to beginning the history (i.e., comfortable room temperature, comfortable position, empty bladder, good but not harsh lighting).

Sit at eye level 4 to 5 feet apart from the patient.

(Keep in mind that some patients such as those of traditional Hispanic, East Indian, and Middle Eastern background may prefer closer physical proximity and may negatively perceive an effort on your part to reestablish distance if they have moved closer to you.)

Avoid sitting with a bright light behind you, which creates glare and makes it difficult for the patient to look at you without squinting or shading the eyes.

Be calm, confident yet empathetic, and nonjudgmental.

Explain the purpose of obtaining the health history.

Reassure the patient regarding the confidentiality of the history.

Use clear, unambiguous language appropriate to the background of the patient. Avoid both use of terms that the patient may not understand and oversimplification.

Ask one question at a time (e.g., "Are you allergic to foods?" as opposed to "Are you allergic to foods, drugs, animal dander, pollen?")

Begin with neutral, factual questions; gradually progress to questions of a potentially sensitive or embarrassing nature.

Ask direct closed-ended questions (call for a one- or two-word answer) to obtain factual information in a time-efficient manner.

Ask open-ended questions (cannot be answered in one or two words) to obtain information about perceptions, understandings, and feelings.

Avoid leading questions (i.e., those that suggest a correct or acceptable answer). (This is especially critical with Asian patients, who often place a strong value on social harmony.)

Allow time for the patient to consider the question, organize his or her thoughts, and respond fully.

Do not "put words in the patient's mouth"; allow the patient to use his or her own words.

Give the patient your undivided attention and acknowledge listening by nodding or saying "Uh hum," "yes," or "I hear you."

 Establish eye contact appropriate to the cultural background of the patient. (Some patients, such as traditional Asians, Native Americans, and Arabs, may consider direct eye contact as impolite or aggressive and may keep their own eyes averted or on the floor.)

Promote accurate, complete communication by using facilitative verbal responses as described in Table 1–2.

Be alert to nonverbal communication.

Validate your understanding of the patient's verbal and nonverbal communication by stating your understanding of the communication and asking the patient to confirm or deny it.

Take brief notes (key words, phrases, times) during the history; do not rely totally on your memory. Do not write so extensively that rapport between you and the patient is lost.

If the patient is hearing impaired, face him or her when speaking; enunciate clearly; use a low tone of voice; speak to the better ear; and use an amplifying or other assistive device as necessary.

Use a bilingual health team member or trained interpreter as needed with non-English-speaking patients or those for whom English is a second language. Avoid use of relatives or friends as interpreters because of issues of confidentiality and lack of familiarity with medical terms. For maximum accuracy, use line-by-line translation, not summary translation.

Geriatric Considerations

Older patients' histories take longer because they have more information to tell. Multiple interviews may be more productive and less fatiguing for the frail patient. Collect the most important historical data first.

Frail patients may be accompanied by a spouse, adult child, or friend. Determine the patient's wishes regarding the presence of others during the health history.

Conduct the interview in a quiet room with adequate lighting to compensate for sensory deficits.

TABLE 1-2 Facilitative Verbal Responses

Facilitative Response	Behavioral Examples	Theoretical Notes
1. Approach the patient with acceptance and genuine respect.	This is best conveyed by facial expression, tone of voice, posture, and attention to the patient's comfort and time constraints: *"What brings you here?"* *"What would you like to talk about?"* *"Would you like information about ___?"* *"Do you have a plan regarding ___?"* *"What do you think about ___?"* AVOID: *"My advice to you is ___."* *"Let me take care of those problems for you."* *"You shouldn't feel that ___."* *"Being afraid of surgery is silly in this day of high technology."* *"Don't worry! Everything will be fine!"*	Acceptance of the person does not necessarily mean approval of all the behaviors, attitudes, and feelings of the patient. It is crucial to distinguish between the person and the behaviors, which may be totally contrary to your value system. Genuine respect is based on the assumption that each person or situation has potential for change. The integrity and the ability of the patient to make satisfactory decisions about life, given appropriate help, must be respected. This avoids the pitfalls of giving advice, being glib, attempting to rescue the patient, or belittling the patient's feelings. Avoidance of cliches and stereotypes is also basic to respect. Reassurance statements like *"Don't worry!"* do not really reassure. To provide reassurance, be trustworthy and communicate empathy and respect. Also, give correct information at the time the patient needs it.

| 2. Reflect feelings expressed by the patient verbally and nonverbally. | "You seem very concerned." "I sense that you are annoyed." "It must be so frightening." "Sounds like you are pretty discouraged." DO NOT SAY: "I understand how you feel." Avoid emotionally charged words until the patient uses them. Say: "You must feel so alone." instead of "You feel abandoned." AVOID: "You are enraged (depressed)." "What a panic you are in!" "You must despise that!" "Are you suicidal?" Instead say: "Do you ever think of hurting yourself?" | Reflection of the patient's feelings communicates empathy and builds trust essential to a therapeutic relationship. Reflection seeks to demonstrate understanding of what the patient is experiencing. It is rarely appropriate for a nurse to say, "I understand how you feel." Only the patient can say, "The nurse understands." Use gentle terms to assess the degree of feelings initially. Once the patient uses a more potent, emotionally charged word, it is appropriate for you to use it. Be aware of cultural and age differences in regard to charged words. For example, elderly American women, often raised to believe that a lady should not get angry, may feel the word "angry" is taboo. Asians may also be uncomfortable with the word "angry," whereas persons under age 50 raised in the culture of the United States, are likely to have no difficulty with it. |

Table continued on following page

13

TABLE 1-2 Facilitative Verbal Responses *Continued*

Facilitative Response	Behavioral Examples	Theoretical Notes
3. Encourage expression of feelings, perceptions, and attitudes by using open-ended questions.	*"Tell me about ___."* *"What were you feeling (thinking) when that happened?"* *"Describe what that was like."* *"Go on."* Wait attentively during periods of silence to give the patient time to organize his/her thoughts.	Use of open-ended questions to encourage expression allows you to learn what is important to the patient rather than make assumptions based upon your priorities. It also allows the patient to verbalize feelings and perceptions and thus begin to identify the cause of vague inner turmoil and to work on the problem. Even when patients already understand the nature of their problems, the opportunity to ventilate is extremely helpful. "Talking it out" is a major stress reducer. It is also true that persons who "talk it out" have less need to "act it out" in socially negative or health-endangering ways.
4. Focus and structure the discussion.	*"Let's get back to what you said about ___."* *"Let's see if we can list the reasons."* *"In exactly what way has ___ been helpful to you?"* *"Let's try to put things in order of priority."*	Focusing brings the digressing patient back to the main discussion. You should listen for themes, even among the trivia. Similarities and differences in descriptions of events or persons by the patient should be pointed out. An overtalkative or aggressively hostile patient may present a special

"Go back to the beginning and tell me step by step."	challenge. It may be difficult to collect relevant data in a reasonable time period unless you firmly focus on one idea at a time. Remember that all behavior has meaning. Try to determine the reason for the overtalkativeness or hostility to reduce or diffuse it. Courteously interrupt with verbal and nonverbal cues when the discussion persistently wanders. Anxiety may make it difficult for a patient to focus on a particular topic for any length of time and your persistence with that topic may impede communication.
"Let's go over the choices you have."	
"I won't be giving you advice but if we carefully look at your options together, I think you will have a better sense of what you need to do next."	
"WHAT happened then?"	
"WHERE was that?"	
"WHEN did you become aware?"	
"HOW did that make you feel?"	Recognize that some patients use symbolic language or vague generalities to discuss anxiety-laden information.
Avoid "WHY?" questions because they tend to make people feel defensive.	Try to help the patient organize what is being said. Often a patient has no idea where to begin to deal with the problems, especially if a number of unmet needs exist.
	Closed-ended questions, worded so that they can be answered with one or two words, are sometimes appropriate in structuring the discussion or filling gaps in the data.
	Help the patient delineate the collaborative role of the nurse and the active participation and basic responsibility of self in his/her own care.

Table continued on following page

TABLE 1-2 Facilitative Verbal Responses Continued

Facilitative Response	Behavioral Examples	Theoretical Notes
5. Restate to clarify, validate, or confront inconsistencies.	*"Am I clear that you said __?"* *"Could you go over that again?"* *"Let's see if I have that right. You said __."* *"In other words, you want to __."* *"Did you really mean __ when you said __?"* *"What about __?"* *"You said __ but now you are saying __?"* *"Let's see. You did __ but you say __. I don't understand."* *"You were smiling when you said you are so discouraged. How come?"* *"Do you really believe that?"*	Restatement conveys a strong message that what the patient says is important, and it conveys empathy. State the implied when the patient makes vague hints. Clarification helps both you and the patient understand what has been communicated in greater depth. Voicing doubts and using gentle confrontation to point out discrepancies promotes realistic thinking in greater depth.
6. Provide feedback, interpretation, and summary.	*"I have the feeling that talking about __ makes you uncomfortable. Am I right?"* *"I notice that whenever I mention __ you change the subject. Is there a reason for this that you would like to talk about?"* *"Let's explore alternatives."*	Feedback should be descriptive and focus on concrete behaviors. It should not be judgmental. Alternatives should be explored, but giving advice should be avoided. The patient should be continually encouraged to give you feedback.

"It sounds like you really want to ___. Am I correct?"

"I would like to review what I think I heard you say. Please correct me if I'm wrong."

"Let me summarize what has been said and tell you how I see what is going on in your life."

"Here is some information about ___ and a list of resources."

"We agreed that you would first ___ and then contact ___. Am I correct?"

"It looks like we've identified the major problems facing you and we talked about how you might begin to tackle them. Do you have any questions?"

"It seems to me that some progress has been made today. What do you think?"

Summarizing synthesizes. It emphasizes major points, highlights progress, confirms consensual validation, and reinforces important information. It may be in written as well as verbal form. A plan for problem solving is mutually agreed upon and a sense of closure is provided.

Older patients' chronic health problems often impact on function. When functions cannot be performed, assess what support services are available to meet the need.

 Pediatric Considerations

Patient Profile Data

Birth child, adopted

Primary caretaker

Past Personal Health Data

Type of delivery

Apgar score

Gestational age

Birth weight

Neonatal complications/interventions

Feeding history (i.e., breast or bottle fed, type of formula, introduction of solids)

Past vitamin or fluoride regimens

Developmental milestones (Table 1–3)

Life-Style Data

Nanny, day care, "latch-key" child

Nuclear family, blended family, single parent, kinship care, foster care

Number of siblings, birth order

Sleeping arrangements (own room, sleeps with others)

Health Management Data

Home safety (e.g., cleaning fluids and corrosives placed in high cabinets, electric sockets plugged, water temperature lowered)

Emergency medical care, poison control telephone numbers available to caretaker; ipecac in the home

Use of car seat or seat belts

Tobacco use by caretakers or others in the home

Preventive dental care

Dietary practices

TABLE 1-3	Developmental Landmarks
Age	**Developmental Landmark**
Two weeks	Lifts head while prone. Regards other's face.
Two months	Grasps rattle. Coos/Reciprocal vocalization. Follows object 180 degrees. Smiles responsively.
Four months	Holds head and neck up to make 90 angle. Rolls prone to supine. Hands midline. Laughs. Squeals. Follows object past midline.
Six months	No head lag if baby is pulled to sitting position by hand. Rolls from back to abdomen or vice versa. Sits with a little support (one hand). Bears weight. Reaches for object on table, raking pattern. Turns towards sounds. Babbles vowels. Smiles spontaneously.
Nine months	Sits alone. Crawls. Pulls self to standing position. Stands holding to solid object (not human). Has pincer grasp. Tries to get toy just out of reach. Transfers block from hand to hand. Resists toy being pulled away. Says "Da-da," "Ma-ma." Initial anxiety towards strangers. Plays "peek-a-boo."
Twelve months	Stands alone 2–3 seconds if outside support removed. Cruises—walks around holding onto furniture. Bangs 2 blocks together if held one in each hand. Imitates vocalizing heard in preceding minute. Has 2-word vocabulary. Waves bye-bye.

Table continued on following page

TABLE 1–3	Developmental Landmarks *Continued*
Age	Developmental Landmark
Fifteen months	Walks well. Stoops to recover toys on floor. Tries to feed self. Uses "Da-da" and "Ma-ma" specifically and correctly. Has 4 to 6-word vocabulary. Indicates wants by pulling, pointing, or appropriate verbalization (not crying). Plays "pat-a-cake."
Eighteen months	Walks up stairs with 1 hand held. Puts 1 block on another without it falling off. Rolls or tosses ball back to examiner. Drinks from cup without spilling too much; uses spoon. Assists in removing clothing. Has 6 to 10-word vocabulary. Knows 1 body part. Mimics household chores like sweeping, dusting, etc.
Two years	Goes up and down stairs holding rail. Kicks ball in front of self without support. Balances 4 blocks on top of one another. Dumps small object out of bottle after demonstration. Scribbles spontaneously—purposeful marking of more than one stroke. Combines 2 words. Has 50-word vocabulary. Points correctly to 5 parts of body. Does simple tasks in house.
Two-and-one-half years	Throws overhand with demonstration. Combines 2 words meaningfully (subjects/predicates). Names correctly 1 picture in book, e.g., cat.
Three years	Alternates feet ascending stairs. Jumps in place. Pedals tricycle. Dumps small articles from bottle without demonstration. Copies circle. Uses sentences intelligible to strangers.

Table continued on following page

TABLE 1–3	Developmental Landmarks *Continued*
Age	**Developmental Landmark**
	Puts on clothing.
	Washes and dries hands.
	Knows name, sex, and age.
Four years	Alternates feet descending stairs.
	Balances on 1 foot for 5 seconds.
	Builds bridge of 3 blocks after demonstration.
	Copies circles and cross.
	Identifies longer of 2 lines.
	Cuts/Pastes.
	Dresses with supervision.
	Plays with other children so they interact.
	Understands what to do when tired, cold, hungry.
	Knows first and last names.
Five years	Hops 2 or more times.
	Imitates forward heel-to-toe walk.
	Catches ball thrown 3 feet.
	Draws 3-part man.
	Dresses without supervision.
	Recognizes colors 3/4.
Six years	Performs backward heel-toe walk.
	Copies a square.
	Draws a man with 6 parts.
	Ties shoelaces.
	Recognizes letters.
	Writes name.
	Defines 6 single words, e.g., ball, lake, house.
	Names materials of which things are made, e.g., spoon, door.

Adapted from Records used by the New City Pediatric Group P.C.

Sleep patterns

Bowel habits

Past hemoglobin, lead screening

Exercise, sports

Type of fun or leisure time activities

Psychosocial Data

Means of disciplining, behavior problems at home or in school

Fears, nervous habits, means of coping with stress

What grade in school, academic performance satisfactory

Trouble with the law

Values re: sexual matters (i.e., in harmony or conflict with parents)

Guidelines for Obtaining a Child's Health History

Provide adolescents with privacy and confidentiality

The Physical Examination

2

TECHNIQUES OF PHYSICAL EXAMINATION

The four basic techniques in physical examination are:

Inspection

Palpation

Percussion

Auscultation

Palpation follows inspection except when examining the abdomen, in which case it follows percussion and auscultation to avoid distortion of bowel sounds.

Inspection

Inspection is the visual examination of the patient.

Guidelines for Effective Inspection

Be systematic.

Fully expose the area to be inspected; cover other body parts to respect the patient's modesty.

Use a good light, preferably natural light, which will not distort colors. Use tangential lighting, which casts shadows, to increase visibility of variations in the body surface.

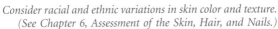 *Consider racial and ethnic variations in skin color and texture. (See Chapter 6, Assessment of the Skin, Hair, and Nails.)*

Maintain a comfortable room temperature, as skin color is affected by both heat and cold.

Observe color, shape, size, symmetry, position, and movement.

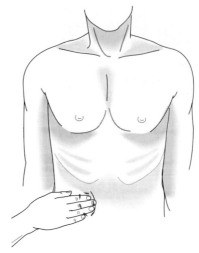

FIGURE 2-1 Light palpation. Note hand is parallel to area being palpated and fingers are pressing down 1 to 2 cm (½–¾ inch).

Compare bilateral structures for similarities and differences. Take advantage of time spent with the patient when obtaining the health history to begin to inspect exposed body parts.

Palpation

Palpation is the use of the hand to touch for the purpose of determining temperature, moisture, size, shape, position, texture, consistency, and movement. It is also used to check pulses; to elicit tenderness, guarding, and rebound tenderness; and to check for distention and edema.

Types of Palpation

LIGHT PALPATION

USE: To check muscle tone and assess for tenderness

TECHNIQUE: Place the hand with fingers together parallel to the area being palpated. Press down 1 to 2 cm (½ to ¾ inch). Repeat in ever-widening circles until the area to be examined is covered (Fig. 2–1). Perform light palpation prior to deep palpation.

DEEP PALPATION

USE: To identify abdominal organs and abdominal masses

TECHNIQUE: With the fingers together, approach the area to be examined at a 60 degree angle and use the pads and tips of the fingers of one hand to press in 4 cm (2 inches) (Fig. 2–2A). Be certain your fingernails are short to avoid injuring the patient's skin and keep in mind that deep palpation can be uncomfortable.

For two-handed deep palpation proceed as above but place the fingers of one hand on top of those of the other (Fig. 2–2B).

Guidelines for Effective Palpation

Wash your hands before and after palpation.

Be aware that touching can cause embarrassment, and attempt to put the patient at ease: Explain all actions, procedures, the "what, where, and why," as well as any expected discomfort.

Make certain your hands are warm before placing them on the patient's skin.

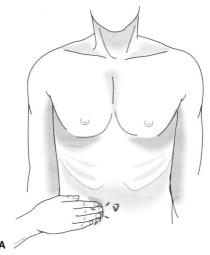

A

FIGURE 2-2 *A,* Single-handed deep palpation. Note 60 degree angle of fingers to area being palpated.

Illustration continued on following page

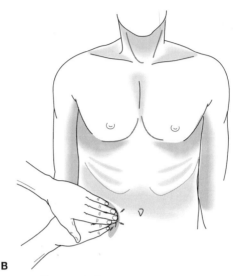

B

FIGURE 2–2 *Continued B,* Bimanual deep palpation.

Ask the patient to take slow, deep breaths through the mouth to decrease muscle tension, which can interfere with palpation.

Palpate tender areas last; stop if pain occurs.

Use the pads of the fingers to assess texture, shape, size, and movement.

Use the back of the hand to check temperature.

Use the palmar or ulnar aspect of hand to assess vibrations.

Percussion

Percussion is the striking of the body surface with short, sharp strokes in order to produce palpable vibrations and characteristic sounds. It is used to determine the location, size, shape, and density of underlying structures; to detect the presence of air or fluid in a body space; and to elicit tenderness.

Types of Percussion

DIRECT PERCUSSION.   Percussion in which one hand is used and the striking finger (plexor) of the examiner touches the surface being percussed.

TECHNIQUE: Using sharp rapid movements from the wrist, strike the body surface to be percussed with the pads of two, three, or four fingers or with the pad of the middle finger alone. Primarily used to assess sinuses in the adult.

INDIRECT PERCUSSION. Percussion in which two hands are used and the plexor strikes the finger of the examiner's other hand, which is in contact with the body surface being percussed (pleximeter).

TECHNIQUE: Place the distal portion of the hyperextended middle finger of the nondominant hand against the body surface to be percussed. Lift the other fingers and the rest of the hand so there is no contact of these parts with the patient's body surface.

Strike the pleximeter just behind the nail bed or at the distal interphalangeal joint with the tip of the middle finger of the dominant hand. Strike at a right angle to the pleximeter using a quick, sharp but relaxed wrist motion (Fig. 2–3). Withdraw the plexor immediately after the strike to avoid damping the vibration. Strike each area twice and then move to a new area. Use only the force necessary to produce a clear tone. Generally, the thicker the body wall in the area being percussed, the greater the force needed to produce a clear tone.

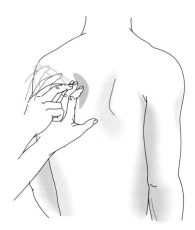

FIGURE 2-3 Indirect percussion.

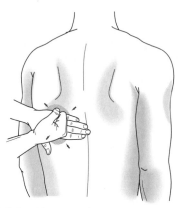

FIGURE 2-4 Indirect blunt percussion.

BLUNT PERCUSSION.   Percussion in which the ulnar surface of the hand or fist is used in place of the fingers to strike the body surface, either directly or indirectly. In indirect blunt palpation the palm of the nondominant hand is placed flat against the body surface to be percussed and is struck by the ulnar surface of the fist of the dominant hand using a quick wrist motion (Fig. 2–4).

Percussion Sounds

RESONANCE: A hollow sound like that produced by the normal lung

HYPERRESONANCE: A booming sound like that produced by an emphysematous lung

TYMPANY: A musical or drum sound like that produced by the stomach and intestines

DULLNESS: Thud sound produced by dense structures such as the liver, and enlarged spleen, or a full bladder

FLATNESS: An extremely dull sound like that produced by very dense structures such as muscle or bone

As a general rule, the more air present in an area of percussion, the louder, deeper, and longer is the sound produced. Conversely, the more solid the area being percussed, the softer, higher, and shorter the sound produced.

Guidelines for Effective Percussion

Ensure a quiet environment.

Have the patient void before percussion of the lower abdomen.

Recognize that obesity can cause sounds to be muffled.

Make certain your hands are warm prior to touching the patient.

Maintain short fingernails.

Percuss from more resonant body areas to less resonant areas (i.e., from areas of more air to more solid) to facilitate detection of tone changes.

Use equal force on all areas to allow for accurate comparison.

Avoid percussing over ribs, scapulae, or other bony structures, otherwise only a dull sound will be heard.

Never use blunt percussion over the thorax of an elderly patient because of the risk of fracturing ribs.

Auscultation

Auscultation is listening to sounds produced inside the body. These include breath sounds, heart sounds, vascular sounds, and bowel sounds. Auscultation is used to detect the presence of normal and abnormal sounds and to assess them in terms of loudness, pitch, quality, frequency, and duration.

Guidelines for Effective Auscultation

Use an adequate stethoscope

- Tubing should be no longer than 12 to 14 inches (30 to 36 cm); longer tubing can distort sounds.

- Ear pieces should slope toward the nose and fit snugly but not to the point of pain.

- The bell of the stethoscope is used to auscultate low-pitched sounds such as extra heart sounds, murmurs, and blood pressure. Hold the bell piece lightly against the skin surface when auscultating low-pitched sounds to avoid obliterating them.

- The diaphragm of the stethoscope is used to auscultate high-pitched sounds such as normal heart sounds, bowel sounds, and friction rubs. Place the full surface of the diaphragm flatly and firmly against the skin when ausculating high-pitched sounds.

■ Avoid holding the diaphragm or bell with your thumb to avoid hearing your own pulse.

EQUIPMENT FOR PHYSICAL EXAMINATION

Basic equipment includes the following:

Tape measure and ruler marked in centimeters
Sphygmomanometer and cuff
Stethoscope with a bell and diaphragm
Thermometer
Otoscope
Ophthalmoscope
Nasal speculum
Flashlight
Tongue blade
Reflex hammer
Tuning fork
Vision chart
Sharp object
Cotton balls
Vaginal speculum
Clean gloves
Lubricant
Materials for cytologic study and guaiac test reagents

CONDUCTING THE PHYSICAL EXAMINATION

Introduce yourself, giving your name, title, and role, if not previously done during the history interview.

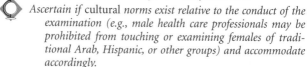

Ascertain if cultural *norms exist relative to the conduct of the examination (e.g., male health care professionals may be prohibited from touching or examining females of traditional Arab, Hispanic, or other groups) and accommodate accordingly.*

Recognize that a patient may feel anxious and embarrassed about being examined.

Act in a calm, confident, organized manner.

Avoid manifesting negative reactions, such as alarm or disgust.

Be sensitive to the patient's feelings.

Maintain a quiet environment free of interruptions and distractions.

Work in good lighting, natural if possible.

Ensure maximum privacy by draping the patient, closing doors, and pulling curtains.

Use Standard Precautions with all patients being examined regardless of diagnosis or presumed infection status (see Appendix 2). Use additional Transmission-Based Precautions if the situation indicates.

Position the patient appropriately for the part of the body examined (Table 2–1).

Promote the patient's physical comfort: use warm hands and instruments and maintain a warm environment.

Keep the patient informed of what you are going to do and why.

Be systematic and follow a planned order of examination.

Work from the patient's right side, moving to the back and left as needed.

Be gentle and warn the patient of any expected discomfort.

Pay special attention to areas of the body about which the patient has current complaints or a history of problems.

Allow time for patient questions.

Document findings:

■ Be accurate.

■ Be concise

■ Be organized.

■ Use only accepted abbreviations.

■ Avoid subjective terms such as normal, abnormal, good, or poor.

■ Include both positive and negative findings.

 Geriatric Considerations

Be alert to impaired vision and/or hearing and adjust communication techniques accordingly.

TABLE 2-1 Patient Positions for Physical Examination

Position	Illustration	Use	Notes
Sitting: back unsupported, legs dangling freely		Measurement of vital signs. Examination of head, neck, chest, breasts, back, lungs, axillae, arms, and hands	Use supine position with head elevated if patient is unable to tolerate sitting unsupported

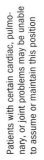

Supine: lying on back with legs extended

Examination of head, neck, chest, breasts, lungs, axillae, arms, hands, abdomen, legs, and feet

Use a pillow under the head and the knees if needed to make the patient comfortable and to relax abdominal muscles; elevate the patient's head if dyspnea occurs

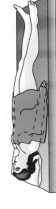

Dorsal recumbent: lying on back with knees flexed, hips externally rotated and small pillow under the head

Examination of head, neck, chest, breasts, lungs, heart, and axillae

Patients with certain cardiac, pulmonary, or joint problems may be unable to assume or maintain this position

Table continued on following page

33

TABLE 2-1 Patient Positions for Physical Examination *Continued*

Position	Illustration	Use	Notes
Lithotomy: lying on back, buttocks at edge of table, feet in stirrups	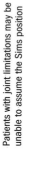	Examination of female genitalia and rectum	As for dorsal recumbent
Sims: lying on side with upper leg flexed in front of body and lower arm beind the body	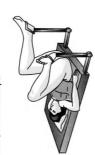 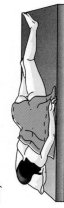	Examination of rectum and vagina	Patients with joint limitations may be unable to assume the Sims position

Prone: lying on abdomen, face to side	Examination of hip extension	As for dorsal recumbent

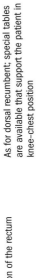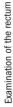

Knee-chest: kneeling with head and arms down to create a 90 degree angle between torso and hips	Examination of the rectum	As for dorsal recumbent; special tables are available that support the patient in knee-chest position

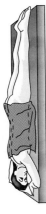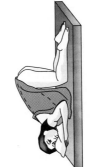

Perform the examination at a pace comfortable for the patient, providing rest periods as needed.

Require as few position changes as possible during the examination to prevent fatigue.

Direct the patient to change position slowly to protect against orthostatic hypotension and/or dizziness.

Be sure the room is warm and the patient is adequately covered because older patients tend to chill easily.

Use a low, wide examination table to promote mobility and prevent accidents.

Never leave a confused patient on the examining table unattended.

Use a step stool to aid the patient in getting safely on and off the examining table.

 ## Pediatric Considerations

Allow the child to stand or sit on the caretaker's lap for as much of the examination as possible before moving the child to the examining table.

Position the caretaker within the child's view; allow comfort measures that do not interfere with the examination.

Approach the patient gently; give firm directions; do not allow choices where there are none (e.g., "Do you want to open your mouth?" as compared to "Please open your mouth now.").

Explain directions/actions in developmentally appropriate language; distract infants.

Allow the child to handle equipment (stethoscope, otoscope) to reduce fear and foster feelings of control.

Save those aspects of examination likely to induce crying for last.

Restrain firmly as needed, the general rule being: restrain the joint above and the joint below the part to be immobilized. Restrain the head by extending the child's arms above the head and firmly pressing them toward the midline.

Provide adolescents with privacy and confidentiality; consider allowing a "buddy" to be present where appropriate.

The General Survey

3

The general survey is a preliminary assessment that provides an initial, overall impression of the patient's outstanding physical characteristics, behavior, and health status. The general survey is begun as soon as the patient is encountered, continues through the health history interview, and is followed by the complete physical assessment.

Areas assessed as part of the general survey are:

Overall physical appearance

- Congruence of apparent and chronological age
- Signs of distress
- Stature
- Body build and type
- Symmetry and proportion
- Facial features
- Sexual development
- Skin color and condition
- Personal hygiene and dress
- Body and breath odors
- Obvious deformities

Behavior

- Level of consciousness
- Mood, manner, and affect
- Speech and speech patterns

Body position and movement
- Posture
- Motor activity
- Gait

Height and weight
Vital signs
- Temperature
- Pulse
- Respirations
- Blood pressure
- Pain

Assess each component of the general survey using the following guidelines.

OVERALL PHYSICAL APPEARANCE

Compare the patient's apparent age to the reported or documented age. Does the patient look older or younger than would be expected based on reported or documented age and knowledge of physical attributes characteristic of that age?

Note any signs of physical distress such as dyspnea, cyanosis, facial grimacing, or diaphoresis. Validate any observations of distress and determine if they are related to a condition that requires immediate further assessment and intervention.

Compare the patient's general height to accepted norms. (See Appendix 4.)

Observe general body build and type including the pattern of fat distribution. Is the patient's size and general shape average, slender, lanky, trim, muscular, or stocky? Are there any evident abnormalities such as poorly developed musculature, inadequate fat, flabbiness, uneven distribution of fat, general obesity, truncal obesity, "moon face," or emaciation?

Note the general arrangement and symmetry of body parts as well as the general proportions of the body and length of the limbs. Ask the patient to spread the arms out to the side and compare arm span to the patient's height. Be certain to consider the decrease in height that occurs in the elderly. Asymmetry of size or shape of body parts, or limbs that are long in relationship to height, constitute abnormal findings.

Observe the size and symmetry of the facial features. Also observe facial mobility noting if it is equal bilaterally. Note any asymmetrical or distorted features, unilateral movement, for example, inability to close an eye, presence of edema, or presence of abnormal movements, all of which are abnormal findings.

 Look for secondary sexual characteristics appropriate for age and gender. Note presence of facial hair, breast size, and voice characteristics. *Be certain to consider ethnic/racial variations, for example, facial hirsutism is common in white women, occurring in 40% of this population and is uncommon in Japanese and other Asian women.*

Observe the skin on exposed body parts, for example, face, hands, and arms. Note color and the presence of any visible edema or lesions. See Chapter 6, Assessment of the Skin, Hair, and Nails for detailed assessment information, including ethnic/racial variations.

Evaluate personal hygiene and dress. Note whether skin, hair, facial hair if present in males, and nails are neat and clean and whether makeup is appropriate. Also note whether clothing is appropriate to weather, occasion, age group, and culture. Note signs of neglect with regard to personal hygiene and whether there is a difference in the attention paid to grooming on one side of the body versus the other. Observe for indications of inability to perform self-care. Ask the patient questions to clarify observations made regarding dress and personal hygiene. Long sleeves or a wide-brimmed hat may be worn to protect against the sun. Oversized clothing may indicate a recent weight loss. Excessive clothing may indicate an intolerance to cold. Untied shoes may indicate pedal edema or pain, or difficulty completing the motor tasks. A belt with new holes may indicate ascites or weight gain. Incorrectly buttoned clothes may indicate a visual deficit. An unkempt appearance may indicate depression or physical illness.

Note any general body or breath odor. Abnormal findings include any sweet, ammonia, or acetone odor on the breath, or the smell of alcohol, urine or feces emanating from the body. Note excessive use of cologne or perfume as it may be used to cover other odors. *Blacks and whites normally have strong body odors while Asians and Native*

Americans have at most a mild body odor; however, given typical American hygienic values relating to bathing, use of deodorants and the like, absence of body odor is the norm for this group. Remember that ethnic foods may affect breath odor.

Observe for any obvious deformities such as amputations, congenital malformations, birth marks, and the like.

BEHAVIOR

Evaluate the extent to which the patient is awake, alert, and aware of the environment. Note whether he or she is oriented to time, place, and person. Note the level of understanding of questions and the ability to answer them and follow instructions. Routine questions posed during the health history usually reveal this information. See Chapter 5, Mental Status Assessment for more detailed assessment information.

Note mood, manner, and affect and their appropriateness to the situation. Compare the patient's verbal responses with his or her nonverbal behaviors. Expect the patient to be mildly anxious but attentive and cooperative. High levels of anxiety, agitation, an angry, aggressive, or combative attitude; inattention, inappropriate affect or responses; apathy, depression, euphoria, or bizarre mannerisms such as repeated patting or rubbing of body parts are abnormal findings.

Note speech pattern, pace, vocabulary, sentence structure, and thought pattern as well as quality, tone, clarity, and strength of voice. Note any speech defects. Consider sociocultural variations such as foreign accents or use of words in persons for whom English is a second language. Speech is normally even and moderately paced with appropriate words articulated in a clear, understandable voice. Abnormal findings include slow, fast, halting, deliberate, interrupted, slurred, or garbled speech; soft, loud, weak, hoarse, monotone, or high-pitched voice; stuttering or lisping; aphasia, dysphasia, or inappropriate vocabulary.

BODY POSITION AND MOVEMENT

Observe the patient's posture while standing and sitting and note the positions assumed. Posture should be relaxed with the body in good alignment. The body should not be bent, stooped, stiff, tense, rigid or overly relaxed. Shoulders should not be slumped.

Observe the patient's movements. Note the smoothness, coordination, and symmetry of movement as well as the presence of any involuntary movements of the face and limbs. Abnormal findings include jerky, uncoordinated, asymmetrical voluntary movements; immobility, paresis, or paralysis of body parts; or the presence of abnormal movements such as tremors, tics, fasiculations, or sudden, bizarre, repeated, purposeless, movements.

Assess gait by observing the patient walking into the examining room or asking the patient to walk a short distance away from, and then toward you. Note speed, smoothness and style of walking, and whether any assistive devices are used. Normal gait is smooth, coordinated, even, and steady. Balance is good and arms swing freely at the sides. Abnormal findings include stiff, staggering, stumbling, unsteady, uncoordinated, shuffling, accelerating gaits; limping, dragging, extension or circumduction of the leg when walking; difficulty stopping, loss of balance, and increased, decreased, or asymmetrical arm swing.

HEIGHT AND WEIGHT

Use a floor model balance beam platform scale to weigh patients who are able to stand unassisted and a bed or chair scale for those who are immobilized or unable to stand alone. Check that the scale is balanced, that is, that the balance bar remains centered when the weights are placed on the zero mark. Adjust if necessary. Have the patient remove shoes and any excessively heavy outerwear and stand centered and unsupported, on the scale, which has been covered with a clean paper towel. Record the patient's weight and compare it with the recommended range for the patient's sex, height, and frame size. (See Appendix 4.) In evaluating the patient's weight be certain to consider ethnic/racial variations.

Measure height of patients able to stand alone by using the sliding, vertical measuring bar attached to the floor model scale or use a tape measure or measuring stick attached to the wall. Have the patient stand straight with feet together, without shoes, arms at the sides, and looking directly ahead. If being measured against a wall, heels, buttocks, shoulders, and head should be against it. Measure the height of an immobilized patient by marking the top of the head and the heels on the sheet while the patient is stretched out in supine position. Measure the distance between the marks. For patients with marked osteoporosis and spinal curvature as well as those confined to a bed or wheelchair, arm span rather than height may be measured. This is done by directing the patient to hold his or her arms straight out to the sides of the body and measuring from the tip of the middle finger of one hand to the tip of the middle finger of the other.

VITAL SIGNS

Obtain temperature, pulse, respirations, and blood pressure using the guidelines that follow. Be certain to always tell the patient what you are going to do, make the patient as comfortable as possible, and use Standard Precautions.

Temperature Measurement

Determine the best method of temperature measurement for the patient and select the appropriate thermometer. Avoid oral measurement in patients who are disoriented, confused, comatose, or unable to keep the mouth closed, and in those who are intubated, have chills, have a history of seizures, or have had recent oral surgery, and/or are receiving oxygen by face mask. Oral temperature also should not be taken for at least 15 minutes following gum chewing, ingestion of hot or cold fluids, and/or smoking. Do not take a rectal temperature in patients unable to follow directions or remain still, or those with recent rectal surgery, hemorrhoids, and/or position limitations.

When using an electronic thermometer, make certain the unit is charged and place a disposable cover over the probe. If taking an oral temperature, place the tip of the covered probe under the patient's tongue in one of the sublingual pockets at its base. Have the patient keep the mouth closed around the probe until the "beep" indicates completion (about 30 seconds). When using a glass mercury thermometer for an oral temperature, cleanse and shake down the mercury to 95°F (35°C) or below. Position as previously described and warn the patient not to bite down. Leave the thermometer in place 3 to 5 minutes before reading.

To take a rectal temperature, place the patient in a side lying position with the upper leg flexed. Wearing disposable gloves, lubricate the tip of the thermometer or probe with a water soluble lubricant and insert gently into the rectum a distance of 1 to 1.5 inches (2.54 to 3.81 cm). Hold in place until the "beep" sounds, or if a mercury thermometer, for 3 minutes.

For an axillary temperature, assist the patient into a supine or sitting position and expose one arm and shoulder. Raise the arm and place the thermometer or probe in the center of axilla then lower the arm and position it across the chest. Maintain this position until the "beep" sounds or, for 5 to 10 minutes, if a mercury thermometer is being used.

To monitor tympanic temperature, gently place the covered probe tip into the auditory canal. Activate the starter and read the digital display in about 2 seconds.

When evaluating temperature readings, consider factors such as the effects of time of day, age, and activity prior to the measurement.

NORMAL FINDINGS	ABNORMAL FINDINGS
Oral temperature 97° to 100°F (36° to 37.8°C)	Fever (hyperthermia, pyrexia): >100°F (37.8°C) orally
	Hypothermia: <97°F (36°C) orally
Rectal temperature 98° to 101°F (37° to 38.8°C)	Fever: >101°F (38.8°C) rectally
	Hypothermia: <98°F (37°C) rectally
Axillary temperature 96° to 99°F (35° to 36.8°C)	Fever: >99°F (36.8°C) axillary
	Hypothermia: <96°F (35°C)
Tympanic temperature	Fever: Hypothermia: { Refer to oral or rectal norms depending on which is selected on the tympanic thermometer
	Chills, shivering, diaphoresis

Pulse

For the purpose of the general survey, the radial pulse is ordinarily palpated. To palpate this pulse, locate the radial artery on the thumb side of the inner surface of the wrist and compress it against the bone using the pads of the middle three fingers of your dominant hand. Release the pressure slowly until the pulse is felt and count for one full minute using a watch with a second hand. Note and record the rate, rhythm, and quality (full, weak, bounding, thready). If the radial pulse is not manually palpable, it may be obtained with the use of a Doppler ultrasound stethoscope.

The apical pulse is auscultated routinely when the patient is known to have an arrhythmia and/or is on cardiac medication. To auscultate the apical pulse, place the stethoscope over the apex of the heart which is located at the fifth intercoastal space in line with the left midclavicle (Fig. 3–1). Proceed as with a radial pulse.

The normal pulse has a rate of 50 to 90 beats per minute and a regular rhythm. A radial pulse is normally full, and

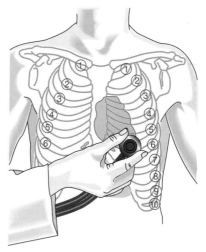

FIGURE 3-1 Position of the stethoscope to obtain an apical pulse over apex of heart at the fifth intercostal space at the midclavicular line.

easily palpated. An apical pulse is easily heard or palpated. Abnormal findings are tachycardia (rate >90 beats/minute), bradycardia (rate <50 beats/minute), irregular rhythm, weak, thready, feeble, or bounding quality.

When obtaining a baseline radial or apical pulse, wait 10 minutes after activity to allow time for the heart to return to a resting state. When interpreting findings, consider the effect of the patient's age, presence of fever or pain, factors such as fear, anger, caffeine ingestion, or stress that stimulate the sympathetic nervous system and factors such as vomiting, suctioning, and physical training that stimulate the parasympathetic nervous system.

See Chapter 16, Assessment of the Peripheral Vascular System for additional information on pulses.

Respirations

Keep the patient unaware that respirations are being observed to prevent changes due to observation. One way to do this is to take respirations immediately after the pulse while continuing to palpate the radial artery. Obtain the respiratory rate by counting the number of complete respiratory cycles (rise and fall of the chest equals one cycle) in 1 minute by observing the rise and fall of the chest or feeling it with a hand placed on the patient's chest or upper abdomen. Count the number in 30 seconds and multiply by two if respirations are unlabored and regular; count a full minute if labored and/or irregular. Note and record the depth, rhythm, pattern, and effort of respirations. Also note any use of accessory muscles and whether repirations are silent or noisy. See Figure 14–6B for rhythms and patterns of respirations.

Normally, 12 to 20 relaxed effortless, silent, regular respirations with symmetrical expansion of the chest wall, occur per minute. Abnormal findings include tachypnea (respiratory rate >20/minute), bradypnea (respiratory rate <12/minute), dyspnea, irregular rhythm, hypopnea (shallow respirations), hyperpnea (deep respirations), asymmetrical chest expansion, use of accessory muscles of respiration, puffed cheeks, pursed lips, or nasal flaring.

Blood Pressure

When taking a blood pressure, follow the specific instructions for the type of sphygomanometer being used. Regardless of type, utilize the following guidelines that are basic to obtaining a safe and accurate reading.

- For a baseline measurement, wait at least 30 minutes after the patient has exercised, smoked, or ingested caffeine.
- Allow the patient to rest 5 minutes before initiating the blood pressure measurement procedure.
- Do not use the arm on the side of a mastectomy, intravenous infusion, or hemodialysis access site.
- Position the patient in a comfortable sitting or lying position with the forearm supported at the level of the heart and the palm facing upward.
- Expose the upper arm by removing any clothing and/or by rolling loose clothing completely out of the way, making certain not to constrict the arm with the rolled clothing.

NORMAL FINDINGS	ABNORMAL FINDINGS
Systolic pressure 100 to 140 mmHg	Systolic pressure <100 mmHg or >140 mmHg
Diastolic pressure 60 to 90 mmHg	Diastolic pressure <60 mmHg or >90 mmHg
Difference in blood pressure between arms <10 mmHg	Difference in blood pressure between arms >10 mmHg
Difference in systolic blood pressure between sitting, lying, and standing positions <25 mmHg; difference in diastolic blood pressure between sitting, lying and standing positions <10 mmHg	Difference in systolic blood pressure between sitting, lying, and standing positions >25 mmHg; difference in diastolic blood pressure between sitting, lying and standing positions >10 mmHg (orthostatic hypotension) Dizziness; lightheadedness; cool, clammy skin

Please refer to Appendix 7 for pain assessment guidelines.

 Geriatric Considerations

Body contours:	Sharpened angles; subcutaneous fat lost from face, arms and legs; fat concentrates on hips and lower abdomen
Posture:	Somewhat stooped as the thoracic spine becomes more convex
Gait:	Speed, balance, coordination decrease in advanced age
Height:	Decreases with age because of kyphosis, flexion of knees and hips, shrinking of the vertebrae and the intervertebral discs, and presence of osteoporosis
Weight:	Gradual weight gain if caloric intake remains constant and life-style becomes more sedentary
	Decreased with very old age
Pulse:	Remains constant during rest, with exercise may take longer to return to baseline
	Radial artery may feel rigid and tortuous
Respirations:	Remains constant during rest; with exercise may take longer to return to baseline
Blood pressure:	Gradual increase in both systolic and diastolic values; tendency to develop orthostatic hypotension

Clinical Notes

Geriatric patients are less likely to develop fever but more likely to develop hypothermia than younger adults.

Obtain an accurate height. Older person's self-report may be inaccurate as he or she may be unaware of height loss.

 Pediatric Considerations

Equipment

Table scale

Tape measure

Standardized growth charts for height, weight, and head circumference

Standardized blood pressure percentile graphs

Pediatric blood pressure cuff

Procedure

<36 months: measure length from the vertex of the head to the heels.

>36 months: measure standing height.

Measure head circumference around the largest circumference of the cranium over the occipital prominence, above the ears, and above the eyebrows. Repeat two more times and take the average.

Measure chest circumference over the nipple line.

AGE GROUP	NORMAL VALUES
Newborn	Heart rate: 80 to 160 beats/minute
	Respiratory rate: 30 to 60/minute
Infants 1 to 3 months	Heart rate: 100 to 220 beats/minute
	Respiratory rate: 30/minute
Infants 3 months to 2 years	Heart rate: 70 to 120 beats/minute
	Respiratory rate: 25 to 30/minute
Children 2 years to Adolescence	Heart rate: 60 to 110 beats/minute
	Respiratory rate: 20/minute
Adolescents	Heart rate: 50 to 90 beats/minute
	Respiratory rate: 16 to 20/minute

NORMAL FINDINGS	ABNORMAL FINDINGS
Upper limits obtained with activity	Upper limits exceeded with illness or pathology

Clinical Notes

Norms for vital signs vary with age and level of activity.

Take the apical pulse in children <2 years; count for one full minute.

In infants, respirations are diaphragmatic and irregular; measure for one full minute at the diaphragm.

Blood pressure can be measured by auscultation, palpation (the point at which the radial pulse is felt upon deflation of the cuff), or use of a Doppler instrument.

RAPID ASSESSMENT

THE PATIENT WITH FEVER

Does the patient have an actual fever?

Does the patient have night sweats? Diaphoresis? Weight loss?

Are there associated symptoms of nausea, vomiting, diarrhea, constipation, dysuria, hematuria, flank pain, abdominal pain?

Is there a fever curve or pattern?

Is there a change in mental status?

Are there associated upper respiratory symptoms—rhinorrhea, sore throat, earache, productive cough, pleuritic chest pain?

Is there abdominal pain?

Are there skin lesions or rash?

Is there uretheral or vaginal discharge?

Physical Examination	Rationale
Check vital signs	Determine whether the patient has an actual fever
Check routine labs	Elevated WBC indicates infection
Check urinalysis	Determine whether patient has a urinary tract infection
Check pancultures on blood, throat, sputum, urine, wounds, urethral discharge and/or vaginal discharge	May assist in determining source of infection if not readily apparent
Check chest x-ray	Cxr may reveal pneumonia, sarcoidosis, tuberculosis, foreign body
Check head and scalp	Note injuries or lacerations, lesions abscesses or infections
Examine the skin	Look for abscesses lesions and infections
Examine the eyes	Fundoscopic exam may reveal findings consistent with infectious diseases

Continued on next page

Physical Examination	Rationale
Examine the nose and sinuses	Look for purulent discharge, masses lesions, sinus tenderness
Examine the ears	Look for discharge otitis externa, otitis media, perforation
Examine the mouth and pharynx	Look for exudates on pharynx or tonsils, strep throat, tonsillitis, pharyngitis, dental abscess decay, peritonsilar abscess
Examine the neck	Look for tender swollen adenopathy. Palpate for tender swollen thyroid.
Examine the chest	Ausculatate for abnormal breath sounds Pneumonia, tuberculosis
Examine the heart	Auscultate for abnormal heart sounds and mumurs, and friction rubs—endocarditis, pericarditis
Examine the abdomen	
Examine the genitalia	Examine the female genitalia for vaginal and cervical discharge, cervical motion tenderness, adnexal masses and tenderness, uterine enlargement and tenderness
	Pregnancy, ovarian abscess, ectopic, PID, endometriosis
	Examine the male genitalia for orchitis, epididymitis, penile discharge and lesions, hernia
Examine the rectum	Examine the rectum for lesions masses bleeding, fissure, fistula, abscess

Nutritional Assessment

4

Nutritional status represents the balance between the nutritional and energy needs of the body for carbohydrates, proteins, fats, vitamins, and minerals, and the consumption of these nutrients. Malnutrition, or an altered nutritional status, results from either undernutrition or overnutrition (nutritional deprivation or excess). Knowledge of an individual's nutritional status is essential to the assessment of the person's general health.

A complete nutritional assessment may not be necessary for each person.

HISTORY AND CURRENT STATUS QUESTIONS

Eating pattern/habits?

Number of meals per day, number of snacks per day, usual meal times, types of food consumed, usual amounts consumed, food likes, food dislikes, eating out

 Consider cultural and/or religious variations (e.g., the prohibition of pork and shellfish from the diet of Orthodox Jewish and Seventh Day Adventist individuals, and periods of fasting among Muslim and Jewish persons)

Socioeconomic/functional status?	Educational level, knowledge of basic nutrition, sufficient or insufficient finances, who shops for food, who prepares meals, adequacy of food storage and food preparation facilities (i.e., refrigerator and stove), eat alone or with others, assistance with ADLs, home meal delivery
Changes in weight?	Current weight, recent weight changes (gain or loss), date of occurrence, number of pounds, over how long a period of time, intentional or unintentional, precipitating factors, content or discontent with present weight, family history of obesity
Changes in appetite?	Date of onset, increase or decrease, over how long a period of time, particular time of day, presence of nausea, vomiting, indigestion, early satiety
Changes in taste perception?	Date of onset, duration, precipitating factors
Difficulty chewing?	Date of onset, precipitating factors or cause if known, description of pain if present, dental history (i.e., dentures, missing teeth, unfilled caries)
Difficulty swallowing?	Date of onset, duration, solids and/or liquids, precipitating factors, treatment, presence of pain and/or hoarseness
Changes in bowel habits?	Date of onset, duration, diarrhea, constipation, pain, precipitating factors, treatment

Illness, surgery, special treatments (i.e., diabetes mellitus, AIDS, chemotherapy, depression, osteoporosis)?	Date of occurrence, duration, type (including recent stress, trauma, extensive dental work), treatment
Eating disorders (i.e., anorexia nervosa, bulimia)?	Date of onset, duration, type, treatment, outcome of treatment
Nutritional counseling?	Reason, duration, frequency, by whom, type, last visit, hospitalization
Special or prescribed diet?	Date begun, duration, medical restrictions (e.g., sodium restrictions), *cultural and/or religious restrictions [i.e., Kosher diet, natural or health foods, vegetarian (type)]*, dietary supplements, cholesterol levels if known
Food allergies/intolerances?	Date of onset, allergens, symptoms, treatment, effectiveness of relief measures
	Consider cultural variations (e.g., prevalence of lactose intolerance among Mexican Americans, African Americans, and Native Americans)
Medications?	Type, prescription, over the counter, starting date, when last taken, dose, frequency, vitamins, nutrient supplements, appetite suppressants, illegal drugs
Alcohol, caffeine, tobacco?	Type, amount per day, frequency, Alcoholics Anonymous
Exercise?	Type, frequency, intensity, duration

PHYSICAL EXAMINATION

Equipment

Floor model platform scale with height measuring attachment

Tape measure

Stethoscope

Sphygmomanometer and cuff

Watch with a second hand

Skinfold calipers

Tongue blade

Penlight

Paper

Pen

Procedures, Techniques, and Findings

1. **Determine the nutritional adequacy of the dietary intake**

   Ask the patient to recall all the food and fluids consumed in the past 24 hours

   Instruct the patient to include the types, and amounts of foods as well as sauces and methods of preparation

   Ask the patient if this is a typical day

   Compare the reported intake to the recommendations for food consumption set forth in the food guide pyramid.

    Use the Asian or Mediterranean diet pyramid if applicable to the patient (Available at www.oldwayspt.org)

2. **Obtain the patient's weight and height**

   Determine weight and height as described in Chapter 3, The General Survey

3. **Evaluate the patient's body weight**

   Obtain frame size

   Measure the circumference of the wrist (in centimeters); place a tape measure around the wrist where it bends (distal to the wrist bone); divide the patient's height (in centimeters) by the wrist circumference (in centimeters)

   Compare the findings to figures in Table 4–1 to determine whether frame size is small, medium, or large

TABLE 4–1	Body Frame Size Determined from Height : Wrist Circumference Ratios		
	Small	**Medium**	**Large**
Men	>10.4	9.6–10.4	<9.6
Women	>11.0	10.1–11.0	<10.1

Determine the patient's ideal body weight

See recommended weight charts (see Appendix 4)

Compare the patient's actual weight to the ideal body weight (% IBW)

Use the following formula:

$$\%\text{IBW} = \frac{\text{Actual weight}}{\text{Ideal weight}} \times 100$$

Determine the percentage of recent weight change (% weight change)

Use the following formula:

$$\% \text{ weight change} = \frac{\text{Usual weight} - \text{Current weight}}{\text{Usual weight}} \times 100$$

4. Obtain additional anthropometric measures as appropriate

Measure triceps skinfold (TSF) thickness to estimate the amount of subcutaneous fat content

Consider sociocultural variations (e.g., African Americans generally have thinner TSFs than Caucasians; socioeconomic status is inversely related to the amount of body fat

Explain the procedure and the purpose to the patient

Ask the patient to expose the entire arm, including the shoulder

Instruct the patient to stand with the nondominant arm relaxed and extended at the side (patients who are unable to stand may sit; immobilized patients should be positioned with the arm extended across the chest)

Locate the midpoint of the upper arm by measuring the distance from the acromion process of the scapula to the olecranon process of the elbow and dividing by 2; mark the midpoint on the back of the arm (Fig. 4–1)

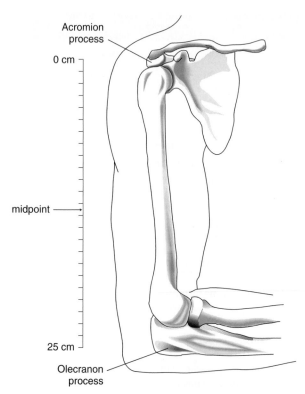

FIGURE 4-1 Locating the midpoint of the upper arm.

Firmly pinch a fold of skin and subcutaneous fat lengthwise between the thumb and forefinger slightly above the midpoint and pull the fold away from any underlying muscle

Place the teeth of the calipers on either side of the skinfold at the marked midpoint (Fig. 4–2)

Wait approximately 2 seconds, until the movement of the gauge stops, and note the measurement to the nearest millimeter

To improve reliability, repeat this measurement two additional times, then average the findings

Record the average finding and compare to the standard measurements listed in Table 4–2

Calculate the finding as a percent of the standard measurement as follows:

$$\frac{\text{Actual measurement}}{\text{Standard measurement}} \times 100$$

Measure midarm circumference (MAC) to estimate both the fat and skeletal muscle content of the arm

Explain the procedure and the purpose to the patient

Prepare and position the patient as for the TSF measurement

Place the tape measure around the upper arm at the marked midpoint

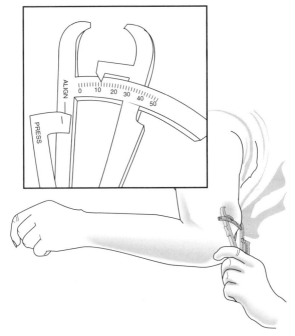

FIGURE 4-2 Use of skinfold calipers.

TABLE 4-2	Standard Anthropometric Measurements	
	Male	**Female**
Triceps skinfold	12.5 mm	16.5 mm
Midarm circumference	29.3 cm	28.5 cm
Midarm muscle circumference	25.3 cm	23.2 cm

Measure the circumference to the nearest centimeter

Record the finding and compare to the standard measurements listed in Table 4–2

Calculate the finding as a percent of the standard measurement as follows:

$$\frac{\text{Actual measurement}}{\text{Standard measurement}} \times 100$$

Calculate the midarm muscle circumference (MAMC) to estimate the skeletal muscle mass and protein stores

Use the following formula:

MAMC (cm) = Midarm Circumference (cm) − [0.314 × triceps skinfold (mm)]

Record the finding and compare to the standard measurements listed in Table 4–2

Calculate the finding as a percent of the standard measurement as follows:

$$\frac{\text{Actual measurement}}{\text{Standard measurement}} \times 100$$

5. **Note any clinical signs of malnutrition such as:**

   Muscle wasting, alopecia, dermatitis, brittle nails, glossitis, cheilosis, stomatitis, bone deformity, abdominal distention, peripheral edema, bruising, tremors, and apathy

   See chapters related to specific body parts and/or systems for detailed examination techniques

   Observe general mental response

   Observe physical activity/energy level

Observe for edema

Observe musculoskeletal development

Inspect condition of hair, skin, nails, lips, tongue, gums, teeth, and eyes

Check tendon reflexes, balance, vibration, and position sense

Palpate the thyroid gland

Palpate the liver and spleen

6. **Note laboratory values**

Consider sociocultural variations (e.g., Mexican Americans tend to have higher hematocrits than Caucasians; serum cholesterol levels tend to be high in African American women and Russian Americans; American Eskimos have a high incidence of iron deficiency anemia)

Review the patient's laboratory data to determine the following values:

Hemoglobin

Hematocrit

RBC indices

Serum electrolytes

Serum glucose

Serum lipids

Serum albumin

Total protein

Urinary creatinine excretion

Serum transferrin

Serum iron

Serum ferritin

Total lymphocyte count

Total iron binding capacity

Vitamin levels

Mineral levels

NORMAL FINDINGS	**ABNORMAL FINDINGS**

Nutritional intake

Food and fluid consumption is adequate and well balanced according to established guidelines	Food and fluid consumption is inadequate or excessive according to established guidelines

Weight

Weight within desired range for sex, age, and height	Underweight: 10 to 15% below IBW (85 to 90% IBW)
Weight within 10% of IBW	Emaciated (undernutrition): >15% below IBW (<85% IBW)
Weight change less than 10% in a 6-month period	Overweight: 10 to 20% above IBW (110 to 120% IBW)
	Obesity (overnutrition): >20% above IBW (>120% IBW)
	Unintentional weight change >10% in a 6-month period

Triceps skinfold (TSF)

Values within 10% of standard reference	Values >10% below standard reference (undernutrition, caloric deprivation)
	Values >10% above standard reference (overnutrition, excess caloric intake)

Midarm circumference (MAC)

Values within 10% of standard reference	Values >10% below the standard reference (undernutrition)

Midarm muscle circumference (MAMC)

Values within 10% of standard reference	Values >10% below the standard reference (undernutrition)

Clinical signs

General mental response
Alert, responsive, good
attention span

Apathetic, inattentive, listless,
confused, disoriented,
irritable

Physical activity level
Energetic, vigorous, sleeps
well

Tired, fatigued, lethargic,
weak, sleep disturbances

Edema
Absence of peripheral edema
and ascites

Edema of feet, ankles, and/or
legs, ascites

Muskuloskeletal development
Firm, developed muscles,
good muscle tone, good
posture, absence of skeletal
deformities

Poorly developed muscles,
flaccidity, muscle wasting,
muscle weakness, poor
posture, bowed legs, bone
tenderness

Hair
Shiny hair, firmly rooted

Thin, dull, dry, brittle hair,
falls out easily, decreased
pigment

Skin
Skin smooth, slightly moist,
color good, absence of lesions

Skin pale, cyanosis, jaundice,
rough, dry, bumpy, scaly,
cracked, poor turgor, striae,
dark circles under the eyes,
echymosis, petechiae,
intolerance to cold

Nails
Nails firm, pink, smooth

Nails soft, pale, spoon shaped,
ridged

Lips
Lips smooth, moist, pink

Lips dry, chapped, cracked,
swollen, lesions at corners of
mouth

Tongue
Tongue dark pink, rough
surface with papillae present,
absence of lesions

Tongue dark red or purple,
swollen, smooth surface,
hypertrophy of papillae,
irritated, lesions

NORMAL FINDINGS	**ABNORMAL FINDINGS**
Gums	
Gums pink, firm, absence of bleeding and swelling, absence of lesions	Gums red, swollen, bleeding, spongy, receding, lesions
Teeth	
Teeth free of caries, discoloration and pain	Teeth loose, missing, unfilled caries, mottling, pain
Eyes	
Eyes clear, bright	Eyes dry, red, dull, conjunctiva pale, Bitot's spots
Neurological signs	
Tendon reflexes within normal limits, balance, vibration, and position sense present	Tendon reflexes, balance, vibration and position sense decreased
Absence of paresthesias	Paresthesias present
Thyroid gland	
Thyroid gland size within normal limits, symmetrical	Thyroid enlarged, asymmetrical
Liver and spleen	
Liver and spleen size with normal limits, absence of tenderness	Liver and spleen enlarged, tenderness
Laboratory values	
Laboratory values within normal range (see Appendix 6)	Laboratory values above or below normal range

 Geriatric Considerations

History and Physical Examination

What factors affect diet (e.g., tooth loss, dental problems, decreased smell, taste or saliva, stomach or bowel problems, chronic disease, depression, reduced social contact, difficulty shopping or cooking, financial restraints, multiple medications or drugs)?

Use a level 1 screen (Fig. 4–3) to aid in identifying older
individuals who require further evaluation or who would
likely benefit from a referral to an appropriate health care
or social service professional.

NORMAL FINDINGS

Edentulous	Poor-fitting dentures may decrease nutrition intake, limit variety in diet, and contribute to difficulty swallowing
Height decreases with age secondary to changes in intra-vertebral discs, vertebra, and posture	Self-reporting of height may be incorrect, leading to inaccurate body mass index
Saliva decreases, gastric motility and peristaltic activity slows	A feeling of fullness and constipation may discourage adequate nutritional intake

Clinical Notes

Multiple medications, antacids, and laxatives can interfere
with nutrient absorption; a complete drug history is a
necessary part of an older adult's nutritional assessment.

Limiting fluid intake is often a method older adults utilize to
control incontinence; assess daily fluid pattern for adequate intake.

Decreasing physical activity may necessitate a lower daily
caloric intake.

Common medications can interact with certain foods, affect
appetite, or change the body's nutritional requirements.
Assess medications carefully.

Unintentional weight loss of 5% or more in 1 month, 7.5%
or more in 3 months, or 10% more in 6 months in the
older patient may be an ominous sign of serious underlying disease and must be investigated.

 Pediatric Considerations

Assessing the nutritional status of a child is essentially the same
as for an adult, with the addition of reviewing growth charts for
percentile ranking and appropriate curve.

Level 1 Screen

Name: **Date:**

Body Weight

Measure height to the nearest inch and weight to the nearest pound. Record the values below and mark them on the Body Mass Index (BMI) scale to the right. Then use a straight edge (ruler) to connect the two points and circle the spot where this straight line crosses the center line (body mass index). Record the number below.

Healthy older adults should have a BMI between 24 and 27.

Height: (in): _____
Weight (lbs): _____
Body Mass Index: _____
(number from center column)

Check any boxes that are true for the individual:

❏ Has lost or gained 10 pounds (or more) in the past 6 months.

❏ Body mass index <24

❏ Body mass index >27

For the remaining sections, please ask the individual which of the statements (if any) is true for him or her and place a check by each that applies.

Eating Habits

❏ Does not have enough food to eat each day

❏ Usually eats alone

❏ Does not eat anything on one or more days each month

❏ Has poor appetite

❏ Is on a special diet

❏ Eats vegetables two or fewer times daily

❏ Eats milk or milk products once or not at all daily

❏ Eats fruit or drinks fruit juice once or not at all daily

❏ Eats breads, cereals, pasta, rice, or other grains five or fewer times daily

FIGURE 4-3 Level 1 screen.

❑ Has difficulty chewing or swallowing

❑ Has more than one alcoholic drink per day (if woman) more than two drinks per day (if man)

❑ Has pain in mouth, teeth, or gums

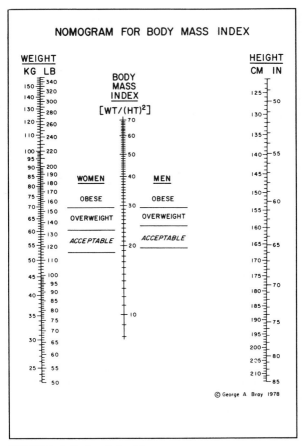

FIGURE 4-3 *Continued.* Level 1 screen.

Illustration continued on following page.

A physician should be contacted if the individual has gained or lost 10 pounds unexpectedly or without intending to during the past 6 months. A physician should also be notified if the individual's body mass index is above 27 or below 24.

Living Environment

❏ Lives on an income of less than $6000 per year (per individual in the household)

❏ Lives alone

❏ Is housebound

❏ Is concerned about home security

❏ Lives in a home with inadequate heating or cooling

❏ Does not have a stove and/or refrigerator

❏ Is unable or prefers not to spend money on food (<$25–30 per person spent on food each week)

Functional Status

Usually or always needs assistance with (check each that apply):

❏ Bathing

❏ Dressing

❏ Grooming

❏ Toileting

❏ Eating

❏ Walking or moving about

❏ Traveling (outside the home)

❏ Preparing food

❏ Shopping for food or other necessities

If you have checked one or more statements on this screen, the individual you have interviewed may be at risk for poor nutritional status. Please refer this individual to the appropriate health care or social service professional in your area. For example, a dietitian should be contacted for problems with selecting, preparing, or eating a healthy diet, or a dentist if the individual experiences pain or difficulty when chewing or swallowing. Those individuals whose income, lifestyle, or functional status may endanger their nutritional and overall health should be referred to available community services: home-delivered meals, congregate meal programs, transportation services, counseling services (alcohol abuse, depression, bereavement, etc.), home health care agencies, day care programs, etc.

Please repeat this screen at least once a year—sooner if the individual has a major change in his or her health, income, immediate family (e.g., spouse dies), or functional status.

FIGURE 4–3 *Continued.* Level 1 screen.

Mental Status Assessment

5

The assessment of an individual's mental status focuses on cognitive functioning and the emotional status of the patient. The examination includes a description of the patient's general appearance, level of consciousness, orientation, communication and language functioning, mood, memory, ability to concentrate, judgment, general intellectual ability, and thought processes. Much of this information can be obtained from general interaction with the patient during the health history interview and physical examination from observation and conversation. Knowledge and awareness of the patient's age, educational background, sociocultural factors, and communication barriers (such as English as a second language and aphasia) are essential to the accurate and valid assessment of mental status.

HISTORY AND CURRENT STATUS QUESTIONS

Head injury?	Description, date of occurrence, symptoms, residual effects
Stroke (CVA)?	Date of occurrence, symptoms, treatment, residual effects
Headaches?	Location, description of pain, frequency, constant or recurrent, time of onset, duration, precipitating factors, associated factors,

	relief measures utilized, effectiveness of relief measures
Seizures?	Onset, cause if known, type, aura, loss of consciousness, incontinence, time of last seizure, treatment
Changes in memory?	Onset, long-term memory, short-term memory, loss of memory
Changes in speech?	Onset, type, cause if known, treatment
Mood?	Onset, duration, intensity, steady, changing, swings
Mental health counseling?	Duration, frequency, reason, by whom, type, last visit, hospitalization
Alcoholism?	Date of onset, duration, treatment, Alcoholics Anonymous
Medications?	Type (sedatives, hypnotics, antianxiety, antidepressant, antipsychotic, analgesics, stimulants), date first used, frequency, duration, effectiveness
	Use of illegal drugs
Educational background?	Last grade completed, high school, college

PHYSICAL EXAMINATION
Equipment

Pencil
Paper
Reading material

Procedures, Techniques, and Findings

1. **Note the patient's general appearance, including personal hygiene and dress, manner and affect, facial expressions, posture, and motor activity**

   Consider sociocultural factors, such as variations in manner of dress

   See Chapter 3, The General Survey

2. **Note the level of consciousness**

   Check arousability

   Observe whether the patient is fully awake

   If the patient is asleep or unconscious, call the patient by name in an increasingly loud voice

   If there is no response, continue to increase the stimulus by touching the arm, gently shaking the shoulder, or producing a painful stimulus as necessary until a response is elicited

   Apply a painful stimulus by pressing on the base of the thumb nailbed

   Terminate the painful stimulus as soon as a response is noted

   Check motor responses

   Ask the patient to open his or her eyes or squeeze your hand

   Observe the motor response to a painful stimulus if necessary

3. **Note orientation**

   Determine the patient's orientation to time, place, and person during the course of the interview and conversation

   Check awareness of time

   If necessary, ask the patient to state the correct date, including the day, month, and year

   Check awareness of place

   If necessary, ask the patient to state the name of the hospital or health care facility, or home address

Check awareness of person

If necessary, ask the patient to state his or her full name, age, or the name of a significant other who is present

Check awareness of situation

If necessary, ask the patient to describe what has occurred relative to the present illness

4. Note communication and language function

Consider sociocultural variables such as English as a second language and culturally specific dialects

Check ability to speak

Observe clarity, quality, rate, inflection and quantity of speech

Observe whether speech is spontaneous or hesitant

Observe whether patient uses full sentences, phrases, and appropriate words

Observe whether speech pattern is organized

Ask the patient to repeat one or two words or phrases

Check ability to understand

Determine the patient's ability to understand questions and instructions during the course of the interview and conversation

If necessary, ask the patient to follow simple commands such as to stick out his or her tongue or to touch his or her ear

If necessary, point to at least five familiar objects and ask the patient to identify them by name

If necessary, name objects and ask the patient to point to them

Check ability to write

Ask the patient to write his or her name and a simple sentence

Check ability to read

Ask the patient to read a simple sentence aloud

5. Note mood

Observe affect throughout the course of the interview and conversation

Ask the patient how he or she is feeling

Ask the patient what his or her future plans are

If necessary, ask the patient if he or she ever thinks about hurting himself or herself, or that life is no longer worth living

6. Note memory

Test remote (long-term) memory

Ask the patient questions about past events that can be validated, such as dates of anniversaries or historical events

Test recent (short-term) memory

Ask the patient to recall a mutually known event that occurred earlier in the day or within the previous 24 hours

Test immediate (recall) memory

Give the patient two or three common objects to remember; ask the patient to list them 5 to 10 minutes later

7. Note ability to concentrate

Observe the patient's ability to focus and attend to conversation and tasks

Test attention span

Ask the patient to repeat a series of five or six digits forward and then backward

< and / or >

Ask the patient to subtract 7 from 100, then to continue subtracting 7 from each answer (stop after 5 subtractions)

< and / or >

Ask the patient to spell the word WORLD backward

Test abstract thinking

Consider sociocultural variables (e.g., the interpretation of certain proverbs may be culturally dependent)

Ask the patient to explain a proverb such as "A stitch in time saves nine," or "The early bird catches the worm"

Ask the patient to explain why similar items are alike (e.g., a pear and a banana)

8. Note judgment

Ask the patient questions such as "What would you do if there was a fire in the wastebasket?"

9. **Note intellectual ability**

Test general knowledge

Ask the patient general knowledge questions such as "Who is the president of the United States?", "What is the capital of France?", "What are the four seasons of the year?", and "What are the names of two oceans?"

Test vocabulary

Consider sociocultural variables such as English as a second language

Observe the patient's use of vocabulary during the course of conversation

Ask the patient to define vocabulary words, beginning with the least difficult and progressing to the most difficult words

Test calculation ability

Ask the patient to mentally perform simple arithmetic problems involving the four basic operations (addition, subtraction, multiplication, and division)

Ask the patient to solve a simple problem, such as "How much change will you receive from $1.00 after purchasing two items that cost $.30 each?"

10. **Note thought process and content**

Observe verbal and nonverbal communication for thought process and content during the course of conversation

If necessary ask the patient questions to gain further insight into abnormalities of content and/or perceptions

NORMAL FINDINGS	ABNORMAL FINDINGS
General Appearance	

See Chapter 3, The General Survey

Level of Consciousness

Arousability	
Awake, alert, readily aroused	Not fully alert, drowsy, lethargic, stuporous, comatose
Responsive to minimal external stimuli	Difficult to arouse

Motor response

Follows commands	Reduced or slowed response
Responds appropriately and quickly	Responds only to shaking or painful stimulation, purposeful or nonpurposeful responses
	No motor response to painful stimuli

Orientation

Oriented and aware of time, place, and person	Disoriented, unaware of time, place, and/or person

Communication and language function

Ability to speak

Speech is clear, smooth, understandable, moderately paced, spontaneous and effortless	Speech is unclear, difficult to understand, fast, slow, loud, soft, hesitant, monotone, slurred
Normal volume, pitch, quantity	Speaks minimally, excessively, only in response to questions
Uses full sentences, appropriate and relevant *choice of words consistent with cultural background*	Uses incomplete sentences, inappropriate choice of words, misuse of words
Organized speech patterns	Disorganized speech patterns
Correctly repeats words and phrases	Unable to repeat words and phrases, substitutes words, creates words

Ability to understand

Understands questions and responds appropriately and readily	Unable to respond to questions appropriately
	Responds slowly
Follows instructions and correctly performs commands	Unable to follow instructions and perform commands
Correctly identifies and names familiar objects	Unable to identify familiar objects by name, identifies function
Correctly points out selected objects	Unable to point out selected objects

NORMAL FINDINGS	ABNORMAL FINDINGS
Ability to write	
Correctly writes his or her name and a simple sentence	Unable to write his or her name or sentence
Ability to read	
Correctly reads a sentence aloud	Unable to read

Mood

Mood and affect are appropriate to situation and discussion	Flat, inappropriate affect
Even mood and affect	Euphoria, hopelessness, depression, indifference, withdrawn, extreme anger, hostility, severe anxiety
	Emotional lability
	Use of drugs and/or alcohol

Memory

Remote memory	
Recalls remote events readily and accurately	Unable to recall remote events
	Makes up answers
Recent memory	
Recalls events of the day clearly	Unable to recall events of the day
Immediate memory	
Repeats stated objects completely and accurately	Unable to recall stated objects

Concentration

Remains focused, completes thoughts and activities	Easily distracted, fidgets
Attention span	
Repeats a series of digits forward and backward, repeatedly subtracts the number 7 from 100, and spells WORLD backward, effortlessly, quickly and accurately	Unable to repeat a series of digits, repeatedly subtract 7 from 100, and/or spell WORLD backward

Abstract thinking Interprets and explains proverb accurately	Unable to explain proverb and/or to identify similarities
Identifies and explains similarities accurately	

Judgment

Accurately interprets the situation and draws logical conclusions	Unable to interpret the situation and draw logical conclusions
Expresses thoughts clearly	

Intellectual ability

General knowledge Correctly answers general knowledge questions	Unable to answer questions
Vocabulary Vocabulary use is appropriate for age, educational level, and cultural background	Inappropriate use of vocabulary
Able to define selected words	Unable to define selected words
Calculation ability Completes mental calculations with few errors	Unable to perform mental calculations accurately
Able to solve problem correctly	Unable to solve problem

Thought process and content

Thoughts expressed are clear, complete, organized, logical, connected, relevant, and flow freely	Thoughts expressed are incoherent, illogical, incomplete, irrelevant, and confusing
	Flight of ideas
Content and perceptions are based in reality	Content and/or perceptions are not reality based
	Obsession, phobia, delusions, hallucinations

Clinical Notes

The Glasgow Coma Scale may be used as an additional objective assessment tool to evaluate level of consciousness. See page 80.

Geriatric Considerations

Hearing and vision loss can cause an inaccurate assessment of orientation. Be sure hearing aids and glasses are in place.

Older adults have more potential for loss. Grief and depression can affect mental status.

Response to questions slows with age. Allow adequate response time.

Confusion is not a normal aging change. If confusion is present, determine whether symptoms have developed rapidly or progressed gradually over time.

Pediatric Considerations

History

Is there age appropriate interaction:

NEWBORN: Bonding with primary caretaker?

INFANT: Recognizes strangers, demonstrates stranger anxiety?

TODDLER: Parallel play?

PRESCHOOL: Cooperative play?

SCHOOL-AGE: Group activities?

ADOLESCENT: Dating, interest in the opposite sex?

Maternal substance abuse during pregnancy?

Any developmental delay?

Any chronic illness affecting socialization and/or school attendance?

Recent emotional trauma, conflicts at home?

Physical Examination

The Denver Developmental Testing Kit or other acceptable tool is used for evaluating developmental milestones.

NORMAL FINDINGS	ABNORMAL FINDINGS
Newborn	
Lusty cry	
One fussy period that occurs at approximately the same time each 24 hours; self-limiting in nature	Weak cry High-pitched cry
Colic; frequent crying in otherwise normal baby	
Infant and Child	
	Autism: little or no interaction with others; appears to be responding to inner stimuli; normal IQ
	Attention deficit disorder: impulsive, short attention span that interferes with learning
Adolescent	
Testing limits	
Experimenting with substance abuse	Addiction
Experimenting with sexual activity	Promiscuity

RAPID ASSESSMENT

THE PATIENT WITH CHANGE IN MENTAL STATUS

Is the patient breathing?

Does the patient have a pulse?

Is the patient conscious (assess as per Glasgow coma scale pg. 80)?

Can the patient follow commands?

Can the patient speak?

Can the patient communicate appropriately?

Is patient's thought pattern appropriate?

Is speech altered (i.e., slurred or hesitant speech)?

Does the patient have papillary responses?

Did patient involuntarily urinate?

Did patient have tremors or abnormal movements?

Can patient move all extremities at will?

Does patient have symmetric muscle strength?

Does patient have sensory deficits?

Are the cranial nerves I-XII intact?

Assess the heart rate and rhythm.

Assess lungs—are there normal breath sounds?

Assess the abdomen for distention, bowel sounds, pain, rebound tenderness.

Perform a rectal exam and assess for melena or bright red blood per rectum.

Physical Examination	Rationale
Check vital signs	Fever, high or low blood pressure, heart rates, respiratory rates, or pain can contribute to subsequent changes in mental status, either by putting the patient at risk for a stroke (CVA), poor cardiac output, or hypoxia
Perform a mental status examination	Abnormal findings may indicate focal abnormality of the brain, such as infarct, hemorrhage, mass, Alzheimer's disease, intoxication, or psychiatric illness
Check the patient's orientation—awareness to time, place, and person	
Evaluate the patient's communication and language function	
Check the patient's ability to understand questions and follow commands	

Physical Examination	Rationale
Check the patient's ability to read and write	Abnormal findings may indicate focal abnormality of the brain, such as infarct, hemorrhage, mass, Alzheimer's disease, intoxication, or psychiatric illness
Test the patient's memory: long term, short term, and immediate recall	
Evaluate the patient's ability to concentrate	
Evaluate the patient's judgment	
Evaluate patient's general knowledge	
Evaluate the patient's understanding of vocabulary	
Test the patient's ability to calculate	
Evaluate the patient's thought process and content	
Examine head and scalp for trauma, lesions, masses	Head trauma may have caused intracranial bleed and subsequent mental status change
Examine cranial nerves for abnormalities or defects	Abnormalities may indicate a focal lesion, or infarct in the brain
Examine muscle range of motion, strength, and sensation	Abnormalities may indicate a focal lesion or infarct in the brain
Auscultate the chest	Abnormal breath sounds may indicate the presence of a pneumothorax, pneumonia, bronchitis, asthma, chronic obstructive pulmonary disease, congestive heart failure, which may be causing the patient to become hypoxic
Auscultate the heart	Abnormalities in the rate and rhythm of the heart, the presence of extra heart sounds or murmurs may indicate heart disease, which may cause the patient to be at high risk for myocardial infarction, stroke, or life threatening arrythmias

Continued on next page

Physical Examination	Rationale
Examine the abdomen for distention, tenderness abnormal bowel sounds or bruits and masses	Abnormalities of the abdominal exam may reveal a cause of an acute abdomen or GI bleed including appendicitis, obstruction, peritonitis, ischemic bowel, diverticulitis, abdominal aortic aneurysm, pelvic inflammatory disease, ruptured ectopic pregnancy
Perform a rectal exam with stool test for occult blood	The presence of bright red blood in the stool or occult blood may indicate an active GI bleed, causing acute blood loss, hypovolemia, and hypoxia.

Glasgow Coma Scale

Variable	Response	Scale No.
Eyes	Open spontaneously	4
	Open to verbal commands	3
	Open to pain	2
	No response	1
Best motor response	Obeys verbal command	6
	To painful stimulus	
	Localize pain	5
	Flexion withdrawal	4
	Flexion abnormal	3
	Extension	2
	No response	1
Best verbal response	Oriented and converses	5
	Disoriented and converses	4
	Inappropriate words	3
	Incomprehensible sounds	2
	No response	1
Total		3–15

Assessment of the Skin, Hair, and Nails

6

HISTORY AND CURRENT STATUS QUESTIONS

Sun exposure?	Amount, frequency, time of day, use of protective clothing or lotion, SPF#
Change in skin color, texture, or moisture?	Type of change, date first discovered, constant or intermittent, frequency of occurrence, associated symptoms, precipitating or associated factors, remedies employed and their effectiveness
Change in hair texture, amount, or distribution?	
Change in nails such as color, splitting, or breaking?	
Bruising?	Areas of body affected, size of bruises, date first noted, pattern of occurrence, precipitating or aggravating factors
Change in mole?	Type of change, date first noticed
Rashes or lesions?	Location, appearance, date first noticed, precipitating or aggravating factors, type and effect of self-treatment measures used
Lumps?	Location, size, consistency, mobility, date first noticed, change since discovery

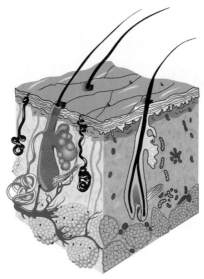

FIGURE 6-1 Basic anatomy of the skin.

Itching?	Areas of body affected, date of onset, pattern of occurrence, precipitating or aggravating factors, remedies employed and their effectiveness
Previous skin disease?	Type, date of occurrence, treatment, residual effects
Skin care behaviors?	Patterns of bathing, type of soap, cosmetics or other hygienic products used, frequency of their use
Exposure to environmental or occupational irritants/toxins?	Type (poisonous plants, irritant chemicals) time and duration of exposure

PHYSICAL EXAMINATION

Equipment

Lighting, preferably natural, strong, direct

Procedures, Techniques, and Findings

Clinical Note

Begin assessment of the skin with exposed areas such as the face, hands and arms. Assess other skin areas as the other body regions are examined.

1. **Inspect and palpate the skin**

   Expose area and clean if needed

   Use good light, natural if possible, since artificial light can distort colors and mask jaundice

   In dark skinned persons, assess color in areas with the least pigmentation such as under the tongue, buccal mucosa, and sclera

   Note general color as well as local, patchy variations and vascularity

   Look for pallor in nail beds, lips, oral mucous membranes, and palpebral conjunctiva

   Check lips, buccal mucosa, and tongue for central cyanosis

   Check nail beds and skin of the arms and legs for peripheral cyanosis or pallor

   Look for jaundice in the sclera, lips, hard palate, and skin.

   Dark skinned persons may have a normal yellow color to the outer sclera. Distinguish this from jaundice in which the yellow involves the whole sclera up to the iris

   Note temperature

   Use back of hand to check general skin temperature as well as that of any reddened areas; compare bilaterally

   Since erythema cannot be seen in dark skin, palpate for warmth to detect inflammation

   Note moisture and texture

   Use pads of the fingers

   Note mobility and turgor

   Pinch and lift a fold of skin over the sternum or the clavicle. Assess ease of movement and speed with which it returns to original position

   Note lesions

   Identify location, distribution, elevation (flat or raised), arrangement, type, color, size, mobility, and type of exudate, if any (Table 6–1).

TABLE 6-1   Description of Skin Lesions

Shape of Lesions

Round	Oval or discoid	Elongated or tubular	Irregular	Ring shaped or annular	Target

Arrangements of Lesions

Discrete (separate)	Confluent (running together)	Linear (in a line)	Arciform (in an arch)	Clustered (grouped)

  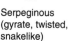

Circinate or polycyclic (annular lesions that have grown together)	Serpeginous (gyrate, twisted, snakelike)	Zosteriform (along a single nerve root)	Geographic

Distribution of Lesions

> Regional–limited to one area of the body, e.g., soles of the feet, chest, or hands
>
> Generalized–widespread over many areas of the skin
>
> Circumscribed–sharply limited to a specific area by a distinct border
>
> Scattered–"here and there" on various areas of the skin
>
> Symmetric–same size and shape on both sides of the body
>
> Exposed areas–areas open to the environment
>
> Pressure sites–areas of increased pressure
>
> Intertriginous areas–areas where skin surfaces touch

Palpate for rashes in dark skin, as they are not easily visualized

Check for edema

Press thumb firmly over bony area of ankle, tibia, and coccyx

Note depth and duration of any resultant indentation

2. **Inspect and palpate the hair, noting quantity, distribution, color, and texture**

   Ask patient to remove wig or hairpiece

3. **Inspect scalp**

   Part hair in several places; look for lesions and/or parasites

4. **Inspect and palpate fingernails and toenails, noting color, shape, contour, surface smoothness, uniformity of thickness, and lesions**

NORMAL FINDINGS	ABNORMAL FINDINGS
Skin	

Color
  General
Pink tones in light-skinned persons; light to dark brown or olive in dark-skinned persons

Flushing, pallor (seen as dull ash or gray due to loss of red tones in black skin and dull yellow-brown in brown skin), cyanosis (only noticeable when severe in dark skin; manifested as dark, dull skin), yellowing (Table 6–2).

Local
  variations
Suntan in white-skinned persons; light lips, palms, nail beds, soles, blue-black discoloration over the sacral area, and freckle-like areas on nail beds and sclera in dark-skinned persons

Areas of increased or decreased pigmentation, erythema, ecchymosis, petechiae, purpura

TABLE 6–2 Common Variations and Abnormalities in Skin Color

Color Variation	Affected Area(s)	Common Cause(s)
Pallor	Skin, hair, eyes	Albinism
	Patchy spots of white on symmetrical and often exposed areas	Vitiligo
	Marked in face, conjunctiva, and nail beds	Syncope, shock, anemia; possible normal variation
	Edematous body areas	Nephrotic syndrome
Erythema	Face, upper chest, area of inflammation or areas exposed to cold	Blushing, fever, alcohol intake, local inflammation, exposure to cold
	Face and upper torso	CO_2 poisoning
Reddish-blue tone	Face, oral mucosa, conjunctiva, hands, feet	Polycythemia
Cyanosis (blue)	Lips, buccal mucosa, tongue, nails	Anxiety, cold exposure
		Heart, lung, or blood disorder
Yellow	Skin, especially exposed areas	Chronic uremia
Jaundice	Conjunctiva, other mucous membranes, skin	Liver disease
		RBC hemolysis
Carotinemia	Palms, soles, face	Excessive intake of carotene-rich vegetables and fruits; diabetes mellitus; myxedema
Brown	"Bronze" skin, especially exposed areas, pressure sites, nipples, genitalia, palmar creases	Addison's disease (hyposecretion of the adrenal cortex)
	Face, nipples, vulva	Pregnancy

NORMAL FINDINGS	ABNORMAL FINDINGS
Lesions	
Freckles, scars, striae	Tracks, varicosities, nodules, papules, fissures, scaling, etc. (Fig. 6–2).
Temperature	
Warm or cool	Hot or cold
Moisture	
Dry	Excessively dry, damp, sweaty, oily
Texture	
Smooth, even, soft	Rough, thick, uneven
Turgor	
Pinched up skinfold returns immediately to normal position	Pinched up skinfold remains tented for ≥ 5 seconds
Edema	
Absent	Mild to deep pitting of skin and underlying tissue 1+ mild (2 mm pit) 2+ (4 mm pit) 3+ (6 mm pit) 4+ deep (8 mm pit)

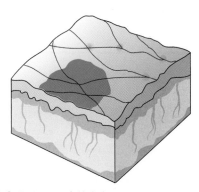

FIGURE 6-2 Basic types of skin lesions.
A, Macule: flat lesion characterized by a change in skin color.

Illustration continued on following page

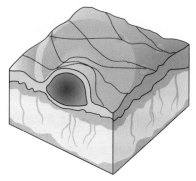

B, Papule: raised lesion < 1 cm in diameter.

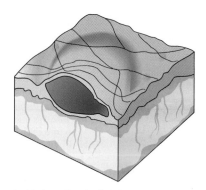

C, Plaque: raised lesion > 1 cm in diameter.

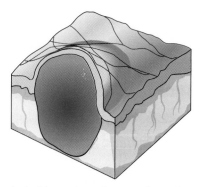

D, Nodule: raised solid mass deeper than a papule or a plaque.

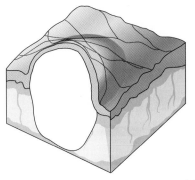

E, Cyst: mass filled with liquid or semisolid expressible material.

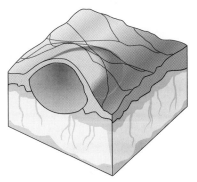

F, Pustule: cavity filled with pus that may be infectious or sterile.

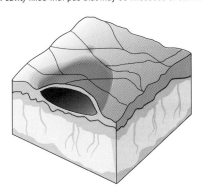

G, Wheal: transient, irregular elevation of the skin due to edema (a hive).
Illustration continued on following page

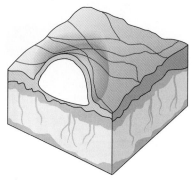

H, Vesicle: cavity containing serous fluid (a blister) of ≤ 0.5 cm.

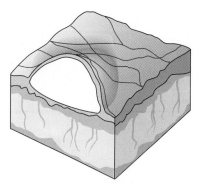

I, Bulla: cavity containing serous fluid > 0.5 cm.

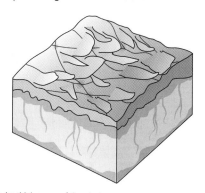

J, Scales: dry thick areas of the stratum corneum.

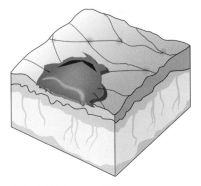

K, Crust: dried blood, serum, or pus residue.

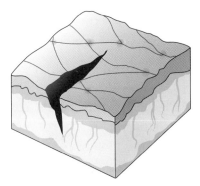

L, Fissures: thin, linear cracks in the epidermis.

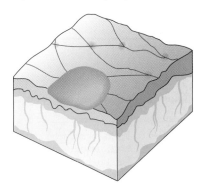

M, Erosion: shallow, scraped-out lesion in the epidermis.

Illustration continued on following page

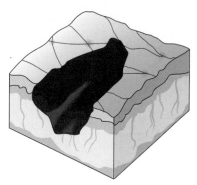

N, Ulcer: open lesion extending deeper than the epidermis.

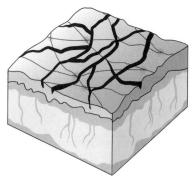

O, Lichenification: thickened areas of epidermis with prominent skin markings.

NORMAL FINDINGS	**ABNORMAL FINDINGS**
Hair	
Varied color and distribution; fine to coarse texture	Patchy or sudden hair loss, brittle texture, absence of hair on the lower limbs, hirsutism

 Little body hair found in Asians

Nails

Clean, curved hard nail, smooth firm pink to light-brown nail bed; *pink nail with speckled pigmentation in dark-skinned individuals;* angle between nail and base 160 degrees

Dirty, jagged, soft, brittle, spooned, clubbed, or flattened nail; horizontal lines in the nail; swollen, reddened, pale, or cyanotic nail bed; splinter hemorrhages in nail bed (Table 6–3)

Clinical Note

Melanin pigment in lips of dark skinned individuals may give a false impression of cyanosis

TABLE 6-3	Common Variations and Abnormalities of the Nails
Variation/Abnormality	**Description and Significance**
Curved nails 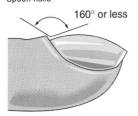 160°	Nails have a convex curve but the angle between the nail and its base is normal Normal variation of no clinical significance
Spoon nails 160° or less	Nails are thin and have a concave curve due to the upward tilt of the edges Sometimes associated with anemia

Table continued on following page

TABLE 6-3   Common Variations and Abnormalities of the Nails (Continued)

Early clubbing

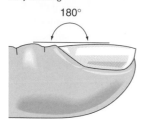

Angle between the nail and its base is straight (180 degrees)

Base is springy on palpation

Late clubbing

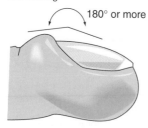

Angle between the nail and its base is greater than 180 degrees because of elevation of the proximal edge of the nail

Base is swollen and springy on palpation

Tip of finger appears rounder and wider than normal

Splinter hemorrhages

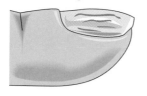

Red-brown longitudinal streaks in the nail bed

Occur in subacute bacterial endocarditis (bacterial infection of the inner lining of the heart) but also occur in other disorders, following trauma, or for no apparent reason

Beau's lines

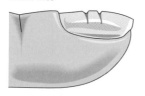

Horizontal indentation or furrow due to impaired nail formation

May be due to acute systemic illness or local trauma

Geriatric Considerations

NORMAL FINDINGS

Skin: Folds and sags progressing to paper-thin, dry, and wrinkled

Senile purpura from minor trauma due to vascular fragility

Yellow and deeply furrowed in sun-exposed areas

Turgor decreased

Veins more prominent

Hair: Thin, fine, gray or white, male pattern baldness in genetically prone men

Nasal orifice, ear, and eyebrow hair coarse and thick

Decreased pubic and axillary hair

Nails: Dull, sometimes yellowed, with longitudinal ridges; may be brittle or have peeling surface

Common Skin Lesions

Seborrheic keratoses: Brown, greasy, warty, "stuck on" lesions found on trunk, face, hands, and arms

Cherry angiomas: Bright red or purple, flat or raised lesions on trunk and extremities

Lentigines: Small, flat, brown macules called "liver spots" on sun-exposed areas

Sebaceous hyperplasia: Yellowish, flattened papular lesions with a central depression found on forehead, nose, and cheeks

 Pediatric Considerations

History

Known allergies

Known exposure to communicable disease, animal or insect bites

Group settings, such as day care, school, college campus

Immunization history

Known trauma

Activity level (e.g., recently learned to walk, participation in sports)

Knowledge or suspicion of abuse

Examination

To check mobility and turgor of skin, pinch and lift a fold of skin over the abdomen.

NORMAL FINDINGS	ABNORMAL FINDINGS
Infant	
Lanugo	
Desquamation	
Mottling	
Acrocyanosis	Perioral cyanosis
	Central cyanosis
Milia	
Erythema toxicum	
Nevus flammeus	
Hemangioma	Hemangioma that obstructs airway, vision
	Port wine stain
Jaundice at approximately 2 to 14 days	Jaundice within first 48 hours and beyond second week
Carotinemia	
None to a full head of hair	
Absence of axillary and pubic hair	Coarse axillary and/or pubic hair
Mongolian spot especially in Mexican Americans	Tuft of hair or fistula over sacral area

Infant and child

Café-au-lait spots: < 3; < 5 mm	Café-au-lait spots: > 3; > 5 mm
	Impetigo: honey-colored, encrusted vesicles
	Bruising in various stages of healing; unexplainable burns or wounds

Adolescent

Increasing pubic and axillary hair	
Comedones on face, back, and chest	Cystic acne
	"Track" marks
Skin alterations such as tattoos, brands	

Pregnant female

Striae gravidarum

Linea nigra

Chloasma

Vascular spiders

7

Assessment of the Head

HISTORY AND CURRENT STATUS QUESTIONS

Injury?

Description, including any loss of consciousness and its duration, date of occurrence, precipitating or prodromal events such as faintness or pain, treatment, residual effects

Headache?

Location, unilateral or bilateral, character and severity of pain; acute or gradual onset, pattern of occurrence (constant or chronic recurrent), worsening over time or stable in intensity, time of onset, duration, precipitating or associated factors (such as particular activities, time of day, or stressful events), effect of movement (such as change in head position, coughing, or sneezing), associated symptoms (such as nausea and vomiting, nasal congestion, or fever); relief measures tried and their effectiveness

Seizures?

Type, sequence of seizure effects on the body, duration, postictal reaction (e.g., sleep, confusion, weakness, headache) and its duration, aura, age at onset, cause if known, frequency, any recent change in frequency, time of last seizure, exacerbating factors (e.g., stress, fatigue, specific activities, omission of medication), treatment, side effects of medication, pattern of compliance with treatment regimen

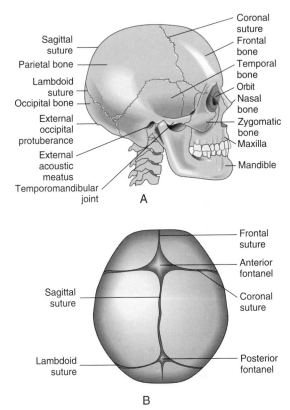

FIGURE 7-1 Anatomy of the skull. *A,* Lateral view of the adult skull. *B,* Fontanelles and bones of the infant skull.

Stiff neck?	Area of neck involved, any limitation of movement, date of onset, duration, constant or intermittent, precipitating or aggravating events, associated symptoms
Facial edema?	Time of onset, location, duration, associated pain, infection, medications (such as steroids), improved or worsened if currently present
Scalp problems?	Soreness, itching

PHYSICAL EXAMINATION
Equipment

Sterile pin or cotton ball

Procedures, Techniques, and Findings

1. **Inspect the head**

   Observe size, symmetry, position, and movement

2. **Inspect the face**

   Observe size, symmetry of eyebrows, palpebral fissures, nasolabial folds, sides of the mouth, movements and facial expressions

3. **Inspect scalp**

   Have patient remove wig or hairpiece

   Part hair in several places and observe for lesions, nits

4. **Palpate the skull, noting shape, symmetry, and inconsistencies (e.g., soft spots)**

   Palpate the temporal artery to check for hardness or tenderness

   Use pads of index and middle fingers; locate artery below the cheek bone between the eye and the ear

5. **Check function of temporomandibular joint**

   Place tip of index fingers on the sides of the face in front of the tragus of the ear and ask the patient to open the mouth; feel the fingertips slip into the joint space as the mouth opens

   Note range of motion, and any swelling or tenderness

6. **Test cranial nerve VII**

   Ask patient to smile, frown, raise eyebrows, show upper and lower teeth, keep eyes tightly closed while you try to open them (Fig. 7–2), and puff out the cheeks

   Observe for mobility and symmetry as these actions are performed

   Press puffed cheeks in and note if air escapes equally from both sides

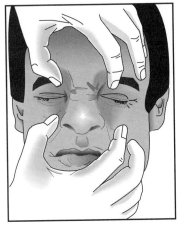

FIGURE 7-2 Testing cranial nerve VII by having patient keep the eyes tightly closed while the examiner tries to open them.

7. **Test cranial nerve V**

Motor function

Ask patient to clench teeth

Push down on the chin to try and separate the jaws (Fig. 7–3)

Sensory function

Ask patient to close eyes

Touch sterile pin or cotton ball to chin, cheeks, and forehead

Ask patient to identify what is felt and where

NORMAL FINDINGS	ABNORMAL FINDINGS
Head	
Size	
Variable	Very small or very large
Symmetry Position Movement	
Symmetrical	Asymmetric
Upright	Tilted to one side

NORMAL FINDINGS	ABNORMAL FINDINGS
Still except for purposeful movement	Tremors

Face

Size and symmetry of facial features	
Variable, symmetric	Excessively large or small, asymmetric, distorted lesions, masses
Facial expressions	
Variable, symmetric	Distorted, absent, or asymmetric
Facial movement	
Freely movable, symmetric	Distorted, absent, asymmetric

Scalp

Smooth, intact, moves freely over skull	Scaliness, lumps, redness, soft areas

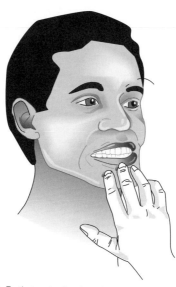

FIGURE 7-3 Testing motor function of cranial nerve V by having patient clinch teeth as the examiner pushes down on the chin to try and separate the jaws.

Skull

Hard and smooth	Lumps, tenderness

Temporal artery

Nontender	Hard, tender

Temporomandibular joint

3 to 6 cm vertical range with mouth open 1 to 2 cm lateral motion Snapping or popping common	Pain, crepitus, restricted motion, deviation to one side upon opening the mouth

Cranial nerve VII

Motor function Symmetrical strength and movement of facial muscles	Loss of or asymmetrical movement Muscle weakness suggested by loss of nasolabial fold, drooping of side of face, or drooping of lower lid, (Fig. 7–4) no escape of air from one or both cheeks

Cranial nerve V

Motor function Symmetrical jaw movement	Asymmetrical jaw movement
Equal muscle strength on left and right sides sufficient to prevent examiner from separating jaw	Unilateral or bilateral decreased strength
Sensory function Sensations of light touch, dullness, and sharpness perceived over forehead, cheeks, and chin	Absent, decreased, or unequal senation
Eyelids blink when cornea touched with cotton.	Absent blink

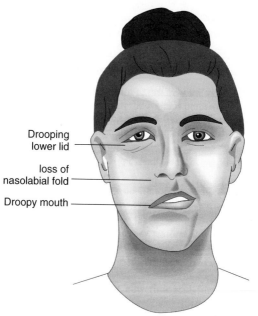

Drooping
lower lid

loss of
nasolabial fold

Droopy mouth

FIGURE 7-4 Signs of cranial nerve VII motor impairment (loss of nasolabial fold, droopy side of face, or drooping lower lid).

 Geriatric Considerations

	NORMAL FINDINGS
Head	Mild rhythmic tremors
	Prominent, tortorous temporal arteries
Face	Nose and brows prominent
	Lower face small with mouth sunken if teeth have been lost

 Pediatric Considerations

History

Type of delivery?
Newborn: position assumed for sleep?
Familial large heads?

Physical Examination

EQUIPMENT

Tape measure

PROCEDURE

Measure the head circumference around the largest circumference of the cranium (i.e., over the occipital prominence, above the ears, above the eyebrows).

Palpate the size and tension of the anterior fontanelle with child upright.

Note the quality of the cry.

NORMAL FINDINGS	ABNORMAL FINDINGS
Infant	
Caput succedaneum: swelling, bruising of scalp over presenting part; swelling extends over suture lines	
Asymmetry and flattening of occiput from newborn sleeping in one position	
Normocephalic premature: increased occipital-frontal diameter; increased bitemporal diameter	Microcephalic Macrocephalic Hydrocephalic with "setting sun" eyes
Fontanelle open and flat	Depressed or bulging fontanelle Dilated scalp veins
Slight pulsation of fontanelle	
Posterior fontanelle: approx. 2 cm (1 inch) diameter; closes 2 months	
Anterior fontanelle: approx. 5 cm (2¼ inches) diameter; closes 12 to 18 months.	

NORMAL FINDINGS	ABNORMAL FINDINGS
Bulging fontanelle *only* when crying, coughing, vomiting	Tense or bulging fontanelle
Molding: sutures over-lapping	Craniosynostosis: premature closing of sutures and fontanelle
Sutures palpable	
Occipital prominence	Dysmorphia: abnormal facies indicative of genetic or congenital syndrome

Child

	Parotid gland swelling above angle of jaw in front of ear
	Erythema, tenderness of mastoid bone

CLINICAL NOTES

Always compare head circumference percentile to the percentile measurements of the previous visits.

Measure the head circumference three times and take the average.

RAPID ASSESSMENT

THE PATIENT WITH HEADACHE

Does the patient have:

- hypertension
- fever
- vision changes
- tinnitus
- photophobia
- nausea and vomiting
- temporal pain
- earache
- sore throat
- rhinorrhea
- sinus tenderness
- discharge from the nose or ears
- sore throat, swollen tonsils, exudates
- intact cranial nerves
- meningeal irritation
- normal motor and sensory function?

Physical Examination	Rationale
Check the vital signs	Headache may be caused by hypertension, fever, bradycardia, bradypnea, or hypoxia causing tachypnea.
Check pulse oximetry	Headache may be caused by hypoxia.
Check electrolytes and routine labs	Headache may be caused by hypoglycemia, dehydration, anemia, and infections, abnormal thyroid function.
Examine and palpate patient's head and scalp for trauma, lesions, abnormalities	Did the patient sustain head trauma, are there lesions, lacerations, bruises, contusions causing the headache?
Examine patient's eyes and vision	Fundoscopic examination may reveal signs of hypertension, diabetes, glaucoma. Check conjunctiva for erythema and exudates (conjunctivitis). Check for foreign body, missiles. Check for injection of the sclera and iris (iriditis). Vision changes may cause headache.

Continued on next page

Physical Examination	Rationale
Examine the ears	Look for discharge, bleeding, foreign body, mass, perforation. Determine whether there is an otitis externa or media.
Examine the nose	Look for discharge, abscess, polyp, epistaxis, foreign body, mass, lesion.
Palpate the sinuses	Tender or infected sinuses (sinusitis) cause headache.
Examine the pharynx	Look for infection, pharyngitis or tonsillitis, peri-tonsilar abscess, dental abscess or infection and decay.
Examine the neck	Lymph nodes may indicate infectious process. Stiff neck may indicate meningeal irritation.
Examine the patient's temples for temporal arteritis.	Temporal arteritis may cause or be mistaken for a headache.
Examine the cranial nerves I-XII	Abnormal findings may indicate a cerebral vascular accident (cva), intercranial bleed, or mass.

Assessment of the Eye

8

HISTORY AND CURRENT STATUS QUESTIONS

Use of corrective lenses?	Date of last prescription change, glasses or contact lenses
	If contact lenses, type and care routines
Vision problems/changes?	Type; right, left, or both eyes; sudden or gradual onset, date first noticed; constant or intermittent; pattern of occurrence (season, time of day); relationship to near or distance vision; precipitating, exacerbating, and relieving factors; associated symptoms (these questions apply to all problems and changes below)
Double vision (diplopia)?	Type (images side by side, on top of one another, or both)
Blurred vision?	Type (objects out of focus, grayness, cloudiness), area of visual field affected (entire, peripheral, central)
Visual loss?	Night blindness, loss of peripheral vision, blind spots (if blind spot, fixed or moving with gaze)
Photophobia?	Severity

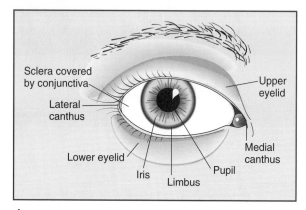

A

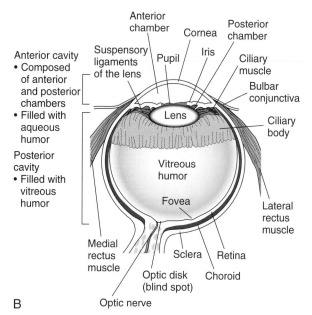

B

FIGURE 8-1 *A,* External eye structures. *B,* Anatomy of the eyeball.

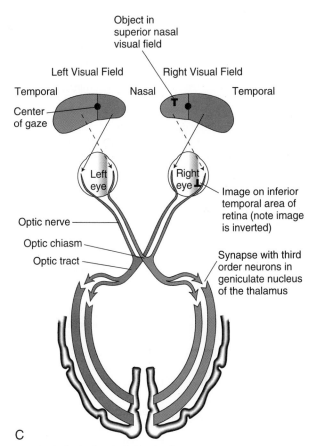

FIGURE 8–1 *Continued. C,* Visual pathways.

Lights/spots?	Fixed or moving, number, color, type (lightning flashes, snow flakes), halos or rings around lights

Eye pain?	Type (burning, throbbing, aching, stabbing); location (brow area, lid, surface of globe, deep in the globe); date of onset; type of onset (sudden or gradual); pattern of occurrence; precipitating, exacerbating or relieving factors; associated symptoms
External eye problems? 　*Redness* 　*Soreness* 　*Burning* 　*Itching* 　*Excessive tearing* 　*Excessive dryness* 　*Discharge*	Type, location, date of onset, type of onset (sudden or gradual), constant or intermittent, associated symptoms, treatment utilized, response to treatment
Life-style factors?	Type of work normally done; type of lighting used; exposure to industrial hazards, fumes, flying objects; participation in sports; use of protective goggles
Previous eye disorders, surgery, or trauma?	Type, date of occurrence, treatment, residual effects
Last eye/glaucoma examination?	Date, purpose, findings
History of systemic disorders affecting the eye?	Diabetes, hypertension, HIV, thyroid disorder, allergies
Family History?	Glaucoma

PHYSICAL EXAMINATION

Equipment

Snellen chart, near-vision chart, or newsprint

Cover card

Pen light

Ophthalmoscope (Fig. 8–2)

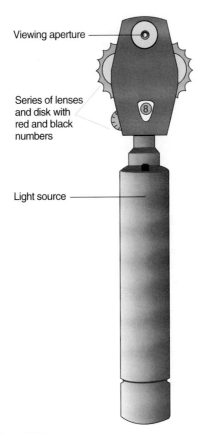

Viewing aperture

Series of lenses
and disk with
red and black
numbers

Light source

FIGURE 8–2 Opthalmoscope.

Procedures, Techniques, and Findings

1. Test visual acuity

Distance vision

Position the patient 20 feet in front of a Snellen chart

Direct him or her to cover the left eye and read the smallest
line of print possible

Record acuity as 20 (distance from chart) over the number found alongside the smallest line of print the patient can read with at least half the letters correct; add to this ratio a minus sign and the number of letters in the line missed by the patient (e.g., 20/30-2, patient can read at 20 feet with errors on two letters what a person with normal vision can read at 30)

Repeat for the right eye

If corrective lenses are worn, test with and then without them. Record CC next to result with corrective lenses, SC next to result without them

If patient cannot see letters, test for finger-counting ability, hand motion, and light perception as described under clinical notes

Near vision (done for those over 40 or with complaints of reading difficulty)

Ask the patient to read the smallest letters possible (with reading glasses if worn) from a Joeger chart placed 14 inches in front of the face

Record results as J1 through J12 (the largest letters) indicated on the chart

Alternatively, have the patient hold and read from material such as a piece of newsprint at a comfortable distance from the face; document in the record the type of reading material and the measured distance held from the face

2. **Examine outer eye structures**

Observe position of eye lids in relationship to the globe

Note any visible sclera above the iris

Inspect the lids

Note closure, size, and presence of lesions or tics

Inspect the lashes

Note distribution, thickness, condition, and direction of lashes

3. **Observe the globe**

Note alignment and position relative to the bony orbit

Inspect the sclera and conjunctiva

Separate the lids between the index finger and the thumb (Fig. 8–3A)

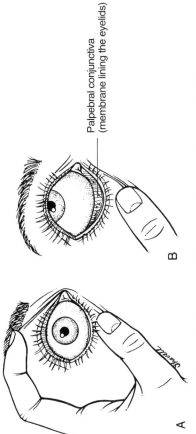

Palpebral conjunctiva (membrane lining the eyelids)

FIGURE 8-3 *A,* Inspection of the sclera. *B,* Inspection of the palpebral conjunctiva of the lower lid.

Ask the patient to look up, down, and to each side

Note color, vascular pattern, and presence of lesions

Inspect the palpebral conjunctiva of lower lids by asking the patient to look up while you evert the lid with your thumb (Fig. 8–3B)

Check the clarity of the cornea

Shine a light from the side onto each eye and observe smoothness as well as for cloudiness and opacities

Inspect each iris

Compare the appearance of both irises in terms of shape, color, clarity, and markings

Inspect the pupil

Note dilatation or constriction, shape, and symmetry between the right and the left

Test the pupillary response to light

Direct the patient to look ahead off into the distance; shine a bright light on each pupil in turn, bringing it from the side to directly in front of the pupil

Observe for constriction of the pupil into which the light is shown (direct response) and for the simultaneous constriction of the other pupil (consensual response); note size of pupils prior to exposure to light, then after constriction (e.g., 4 mm to 2 mm); compare the amount and speed (e.g., brisk or sluggish) of constriction and subsequent dilatation in the two eyes

Test for accommodation

Hold your finger, a pen, or other similar object 10 to 15 cm (4 to 6 inches) from the patient's nose

Direct the patient to look off into the distance behind you and then look quickly at the finger

Observe for convergence (medial movement of both eyes) and pupillary constriction (Fig. 8–4).

4. **Test extraocular muscle function**

   Check for parallel gaze (corneal light reflex)

   Direct the patient to look straight ahead

   Shine a light into the patient's eyes from a distance of 31 cm (12 inches); note the location of the light reflection on the corneas

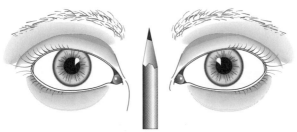

A   Gazing into distance behind examiner

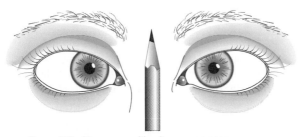

B   Gaze shifted to pen resulting in convergence
and pupillary constriction

FIGURE 8-4 Test for accommodation.

Assess for coordinated movement of the two eyes

Direct the patient to hold the head still and follow your finger with his or her eyes as it moves

Hold your finger about 31 cm (12 inches) in front of the patient and move it through the cardinal fields of gaze

Move your finger from the center out to one of the eight positions shown in Figure 8–5, hold it momentarily, and bring it back to the center

Progress to each of the remaining positions, moving in a clockwise fashion

Observe for parallel eye movement

Observe relationship of upper eye lid to the iris as the gaze moves up to down

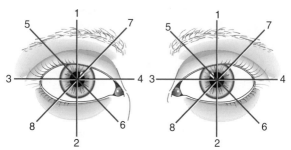

FIGURE 8-5 Assessing coordinated movement of the two eyes (cardinal fields of gaze).

Check for convergence

Ask the patient to watch your finger as it is moved from directly in front of the eye in toward the bridge of the nose

5. **Perform the confrontation test for a gross check of visual fields**

   Position yourself so you have the same visual field as the patient: put your face in front of and on a level with the patient's face; ask the patient to cover his or her right eye and with his or her left eye look into your right eye; and close or cover your left eye

   Bring a raised finger, pen, or other similar object held at arm's length midway between you and the patient, from the right periphery into the visual field in several directions

   Direct the patient to say "Now" when the object comes into sight

   Compare the time the patient sees it with when you see it

   Repeat the above bringing the object into the field of vision from the left periphery

   Repeat entire procedure for the opposite eye

6. **Examine the ocular fundus (retina, optic disk, macula, and retinal vessels)**

   Perform the examination in a darkened room using an opthalmoscope

   Use your right eye to examine the patient's right eye; use your left eye to examine the patient's left eye

Position yourself about 15 inches away from the patient and slightly to the side of his or her line of vision

Select a large round aperture with white light and place the opthalmoscope with lens set at zero diopters firmly under the medial aspect of your orbit and shine the light beam on the pupil of the eye to be examined

Tell the patient to keep looking or staring at a spot across the room

Note the red reflex (orange-red glow in the pupil) and note any areas of opacity interrupting it

Maintain focus on the red reflex while you move your head and the ophthalmoscope forward as a unit until it almost touches the patient's eye lashes

Rotate the lens disk to focus on the optic disk (yellow-orange to creamy-pink round or oval area upon which the blood vessels of the retina converge) of the retina

Locate the optic disk (Fig. 8–6), which is found to the nasal side of the retina, by following a blood vessel in the direction in which it enlarges and has branches joining it

Note size, shape, clarity, and color of the disk margins

Inspect the physiologic cup, including its central depression, and note the cup–disk ratio. Also note the emerging retinal

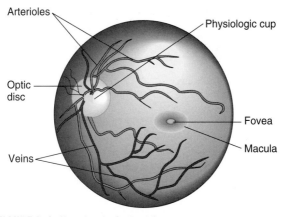

FIGURE 8-6 Normal ocular fundus, left eye.

arterioles and veins (arterioles are light red with a bright reflection; veins are dark red, without reflection, and one-fourth to one-third larger than arterioles)

Observe the branching pattern, fullness, contour, and integrity of the vessels

Proceed to the peripheral retina

Locate the macula

NORMAL FINDINGS	ABNORMAL FINDINGS
Visual acuity	
Distance vision	
20/20 in each eye	Less than 20/20 (i.e., 20/30 or higher with correction, 20/200 with correction in either eye is legal blindness)
Near vision	
J1 or 14/14 in each eye read without moving the card and without hesitancy	J2 or higher or less than 14/14
Outer eye structures	
Eye lids	
No sclera visible between upper lid and iris	Visible sclera above the iris, incomplete closure, ptosis or drooping of the upper lid, erythema, edema, discharge, or lesions
Upper and lower lids completely approximated when closed	
Skin intact and free of erythema, edema, discharge, and lesions	
Epicanthal fold common in Asians	
Eye lashes	
Evenly distributed with an outward curve	Uneven distribution, crusting, brushing the globe
Globe	
Evenly aligned and neither sunken nor protruding	Uneven alignment, sunken or protruberant

Conjunctiva and sclera

Sclera smooth, white, glossy, and moist	Generalized yellow or red discoloration, pallor near outer canthus, cyanosis of lower lid, bulging, inflammation, nodules, discharge

Small brown macules, grey-blue tinge, and/or yellow areas under lids common in blacks

Clear, pale glistening pink conjunctiva, numerous small visible blood vessels common

Pupil

Round, regular, 3 to 5 mm, equal in both eyes	Excessively dilated or constricted, irregular, unequal (Table 8–1)
Difference in size seen occasionally as a normal variation	

Pupillary response to light

Symmetrical constriction followed by symmetrical dilation in terms of amount and speed

Response recorded in millimeters (e.g., R3/1 = 3/1L)	Absence of constriction, asymmetrical response

R = right eye

L = left eye

numerator = resting size = 3 mm

denominator = size in response to light = 1 mm

Accommodation

Convergence of both eyes	Absence of convergence, asymmetrical response

Extraocular muscles

Parallel gaze

Reflections of light on the cornea are on or just medial to the pupil in both eyes	Reflections of light are in different locations in each eye

TABLE 8-1 Common Variations and Abnormalities of the Pupil

Variation/Abnormality	Description	Etiology
Anisocoria	Pupils are unequal in size	Normal in small percentage of the population Central nervous system disease
Monocular	Absence of pupillary response to light directed to the blind eye with bilateral pupillary constriction in response to light shown in the normal eye	Blindness in one eye with an intact oculomotor nerve
Miosis	Constricted, fixed pupils	Iritis, damage to the pons, use of narcotics, use of pilocarpine
Mydriasis	Dilated, fixed pupils	Acute glaucoma, trauma, CNS disease, sympathetic nervous system stimulation, use of sympathomimetic drugs or pupillary dilating drops, deep anesthesia, or cardiac arrest

TABLE 8-1 Common Variations and Abnormalities of the Pupil *Continued*

Variation/ Abnormality	Description	Etiology
Argyll-Robertson pupil	No constriction in response to light or accommodation	Chronic alcoholism, third-stage syphilis, meningitis, intracranial tumor
Tonic pupil	Large, regular pupil with a sluggish reaction to light and accommodation	Normal variation, which is usually unilateral
Cranial nerve III impaired pupil	Deviation of one eye downward and to the side, accompanied by a dilated pupil nonreactive to light or accommodation and by ptosis of the lid	Damage to the oculomotor nerve
Horner's syndrome	Small, regular pupil reactive to light and accommodation accompanied by ipsilateral ptosis and anhidrosis	Sympathetic nerve damage, unilateral

NORMAL FINDINGS	ABNORMAL FINDINGS
Coordinated movement of Eye movement when tracking objects is parallel	Nonparallel eye movement, failure to follow in a certain direction; nystagmus at other than the end point of gaze
Upper lid overlaps iris at all times as the gaze moves from up to down	Lid lag—appearance of a white rim of sclera between the lid and the iris
Occasional nystagmus at end point of gaze	
Convergence Sustained to within 5 to 8 cm	Sustained to less than 5 cm
Confrontation visual field test Patient's visual field same as examiner's, provided examiner's is normal. Noted as "visual fields full to confrontation"	Patient's visual field less than examiner's. Noted as "Unable to detect ___ cm object in upper, outer quadrant of visual field OD" (or OS)

Ocular fundus

Red reflex Uninterrupted red glow filling the pupil	Dark shadows or black dots interrupting the red glow
Optic disk Yellow-orange to creamy pink, round or oval, distinct sharp margins except for nasal edge, which is sometimes blurred	Dark color (seen with eye strain and astigmatism); pale or white color (seen with glaucoma or optic atrophy)
Retinal vessels Paired artery and vein passing to each quadrant, ratio of arterial diameter 2:3 or 4:5, regular decrease in diameter of veins and arteries as they progress to the periphery, mild vessel twisting, artery and vein crossings within 2 disk diameters (DD) of disk, no interrup	Absence of major vessels, arteries constricted, veins dilated, neovascularization, extreme vessel tortuosity or asymmetrical tortuosity in the two eyes, artery and vein crossings more than 2 DD from disk, vessels engorged peripheral to the crossing

tion of blood flow, no in-
denting or displacing of
vessels

Retina
Light red to dark brown-
red with shade corre-
sponding to skin color,
free of lesions

Areas of hemorrhage,
exudate, altered color,
micro-
aneurysms

Macula
One disk diameter (1
DD) in size

Hemorrhage, exudate,
clumps of pigment

Even, homogenous color,
may be slightly darker
than rest of fundus

TABLE 8–2	Common Variations and Abnormalities of the Eye	
Variation/ Abnormality	**Description and Significance**	**Illustration**
Retracted upper lid	Rim of white sclera is visible above the iris	
Ptosis	Drooping of the upper eyelid; may be due to age-related or pathological muscle weakness or nerve impairment	
Ectropion	Outward sagging of the lower lid, which can lead to skin excoriation and corneal ulceration; may be congenital, age-related or due to cranial nerve VII palsy	
Entropion	Turning inward of the eyelid due to aging, chronic inflammation, or scarring; may result in lashes touching globe, causing pain (age effect seen in lower lid only)	

Table continued on following page

| TABLE 8-2 | Common Variations and Abnormalities of the Eye |
| *Continued* | |

Variation/ Abnormality	Description and Significance	Illustration
Herniated fat	Bulging of lower lids and/or inner third of upper due to fat displacing weakened lid fascia forward; occurs most often in the elderly	
Pinguecula	Benign creamy-yellow triangular nodule on the conjunctiva on either side of the iris	
Chalazion	Chronic inflammation of the meibomian gland that appears as a painless nodule usually involving the conjunctival side of the lid	
Hordeolum (sty)	Painful, red, pimple-like area of infection on the lid/lash margin	
Xanthelasma	Clearly demarcated raised, yellow plaques in the skin of the nasal portion of the eyelid; associated in some cases with lipid disorder	
Pterygium	Triangular thickening of the bulbar conjunctiva, usually on the nasal side, which may grow across the iris	

TABLE 8-2 Common Variations and Abnormalities of the Eye *Continued*		
Variation/ Abnormality	**Description and Significance**	**Illustration**
Arcus senilis (corneal arcus)	Opaque white or gray ring around the iris; occurs with normal aging though also is seen in younger persons	
Conjunctivitis	Inflammation or infection of the conjunctiva characterized by increased prominence of blood vessels, redness that is greatest at the periphery, discomfort, and discharge	
Subconjunctival hemorrhage	Sharply delineated deep-red area that slowly turns to yellow and disappears; may be due to trauma, action causing a sudden venous pressure increase, or a bleeding disorder	
Corneal scar	Superficial gray-white opaque area in the cornea due to previous trauma/ inflammation	
Cataract	Opacity of the lens that appears gray when seen through the pupil with a flashlight or black against the red reflex when seen through an ophthalmoscope	

Clinical Notes

Use an eye chart with rows of numbers or E's pointing in varying directions for patients unable to identify letters.

Check the patient's ability to count the number of fingers held up by the examiner if no lines on a Snellen chart can

TABLE 8-3	Common Variations and Abnormalities of the Optic Disc	
Variation/ Abnormality	**Description and Significance**	**Illustration**
Optic atrophy	Loss of tiny vessels due to death of optic nerve fibers	
Papilledema	Engorgment and elevation of the disc with blurred disc margins due to venous stasis secondary to increased intracranial pressure	
Neovascular-ization	Growth of new blood vessels that are narrow, tortuous, and more numerous than surrounding vessels; associated with diabetic retinopathy	
Cotton wool patches (soft exudates)	Grayish white oval lesions with irregular margins associated with hypertension	
Hard exudates	Creamy-yellow well-demarcated lesions that may be discrete, small and round, or large and irregular because of coalescence; associated with diabetes and hypertension	

be read. When 50% or more finger presentations are identified correctly document the patient's performance on this counting fingers test as "Counts fingers at _____ feet."

Test ability to perceive hand motion in patients unable to count fingers. Do this by having the patient cover each eye in turn and waving your hand either up or down or right to left. When the patient correctly identifies the direction of the hand wave 50% of the time, document the results as "Hand motion at _____ feet."

Test light perception if the patient is unable to detect hand motion. Darken the room and direct the patient to cover one eye. Shine a bright light into the uncovered eye at random intervals, turning it off between them. Ask the patient to report when light is seen. Document the patient as having light-perception acuity if 50% of the light presentations are identified. Repeat for the other eye.

Record normal pupillary findings as PERRLA (pupils equal, round, reactive to light, and accommodation).

Document findings in the ocular fundus by noting clock position and relation to the optic disk in terms of size and distance. For example "_____ noted at 1 o'clock, 1½ DD from the disk" (Fig. 8–7).

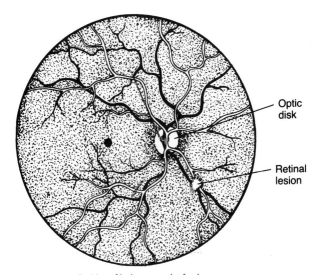

Optic disk

Retinal lesion

FIGURE 8–7 Position of lesion on ocular fundus.

Geriatric Considerations

Additional History Questions

Family history of cataracts?

Date of last glaucoma test?

Problems with night vision, glare, distinguishing colors?

Loss of peripheral or central vision?

Burning or dryness of eyes?

Problems with management of eye drops (if applicable)?

	NORMAL FINDINGS
Visual acuity	20/20 to 20/70 distance vision some blurriness on near vision (presbyopia)
External eye structures	Thin outer aspect of eyebrows due to a decrease in hair follicles
	Wrinkled, baggy lids and wrinkling of skin around eyes due to atrophy
	Bulging of lower lids and/or inner third of upper lids due to pressure of fat on atrophied fascia
	Partial ptosis of upper lid due to muscle atrophy
	Xanthalasma (benign, soft, yellow plaques on lids at inner canthus)
	Sunken because of loss of supporting fat
	Dry because of decreased tear production
	Entropion: turning inward of lower lid
	or
	Ectropion: drooping of the lid away from the globe due to atrophy of elastic and fibrous tissue

Globe	Arcus senilis (white to gray circle around the outer edge of the cornea due to the deposition of lipid and without clinical significance)
	Clouding, dullness of the cornea
	Decreased pupil size and occasional slight irregularity
	Slowed pupillary light reflex
Fundus	Less shiny
	Pale, narrow, straight arterioles
	Increased number of A–V crossing defects
	Drusen (hyaline deposits that appear as small, scattered, round, yellow spots on the retina); may occur with normal aging but may also indicate early macular degeneration
	Vitreous floaters

 Pediatric Considerations

History

Maternal rubella?

Squinting, rubbing eyes?

Holding books near to face, sitting close to TV?

Physical Examination

EQUIPMENT

Snellen pre-school picture chart

PROCEDURE

Check red reflex in all newborns.

Note spacing and symmetry of eyes.

"Cover test" by age 1 year: cover one eye, uncover suddenly and observe for an abnormal shift from a lateral or medial to a central gaze.

Visual acuity test by 3 years of age.

NORMAL FINDINGS	ABNORMAL FINDINGS
Newborn, infant, and child	

NORMAL FINDINGS	ABNORMAL FINDINGS
Variable	Wide-set eyes
Epicanthal fold common in Asians, in whites disappears usually by age 10	Palpebral slant in non-Asian Epicanthal folds
Red-orange reflex	Abnormal red reflex; opacity
Intermittent convergent strabismus < 6 months	Divergent strabismus
Corneal light reflex symmetrical after age 6 months	Asymmetry of corneal light reflex on pupil after age 6 months
Direct consensual pupillary constriction in response to bright light	Absence of reflex
Visual acuity:	
4 weeks: fixation on object	
6 weeks: follows < 180 degrees	
4 months: follows > 180 degrees; convergence	
Dark blue or slate colored iris in light skinned neonates, *Brown in dark skinned*	Absence of iris color
1 year: 20/200; focuses; hand-eye coordination	
3 years: 20/40	
5 years: 20/30	
6 to 7 years: 20/20	
Ptosis	
Chemical conjunctivitis (from instillation of medication in delivery room)	
Small subconjunctival and scleral hemorrhage	

Lacrimal meatus ob-
structed, with tearing
and mucous collecting in
the eye

Pseudostrabismus sec-
ondary to wide bridge
of nose

Clinical Notes

Refer to an ophthalmologist before visual acuity test at 3 years if child has an opacity of lens, does not follow gaze, demonstrates divergent strabismus, fails "cover test," or presents with dilated, tortuous, retinal vessels.

Assessment of the Ear

9

HISTORY AND CURRENT STATUS QUESTIONS

Hearing loss?

Unilateral or bilateral; date first noticed; sudden or gradual onset (if gradual over what time span); general or selective loss (e.g., high sounds, conversational tones when background noise is present); severity; precipitating or associated factors; effects on daily activities, job responsibilities, and social interactions; use of hearing aid, including type and effectiveness

Ear pain or discomfort?

Unilateral or bilateral, date and type of onset, constant or intermittent, type (throbbing, feeling of fullness, dull ache, sharp, stabbing), location (outer ear or deep in the head), changes in the type of pain since onset, precipitating or worsening factors (changing the position of the head, pulling or pushing on the ear, chewing, yawning, or exposure to heat or cold) type and effectiveness of treatment measures utilized, associated symptoms

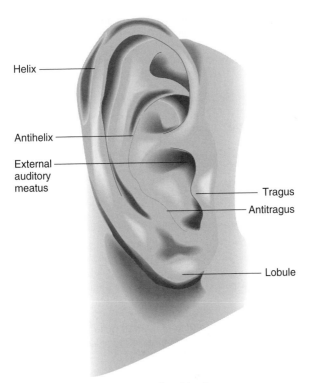

FIGURE 9-1 Anatomy of the external ear (pinna).

Discharge?	Unilateral or bilateral, date and type of onset (sudden or gradual), color, odor, consistency, amount, constant or intermittent, precipitating factors, associated symptoms (skin irritation, canal itching, fever, pain)
Tinnitus?	Unilateral or bilateral, date of onset, quality (high- or low-pitched, roaring, humming, or hissing), severity, constant or intermittent, precipitating factors, long-term use of aspirin or other salicylates (how much, how often, for how long)

Vertigo?	Time and type of onset, severity, constant or intermittent, associated symptoms (nausea, vomiting, ataxia), precipitating factors, type and effectiveness of relief measures used
	Be certain to differentiate vertigo, in which the room is perceived as moving around, from dizziness, in which the patient feels he or she is moving
Last hearing examination?	Date, type, reason for, by whom, results
Use of a hearing aid or other assistive devices?	Type of device used, consistency of use, perceived effectiveness, care of device, difficulties with the device
Prior ear problems?	Type (surgery, trauma, infections, etc.) date(s), treatment, residual effects
Exposure to ototoxic factors?	Use of medications such as aspirin, gentomicin and other aminoglycosides, quinine, ethycrinic acid, furosemide and vancomycin
	Long-term exposure to loud noise (e.g., from traffic, machinery, gunshots, radios, concerts)
Related health problems?	Allergies; colds; sinus, eye, mouth, teeth, jaw, or throat problems; recent head trauma
Self-care routines related to the ear?	Hygienic practices, use of protective head phones or ear plugs

PHYSICAL EXAMINATION

Equipment

Otoscope (Fig. 9–2) with fresh batteries so white, not yellow light is produced

Tuning fork (512 or 1024 Hz)

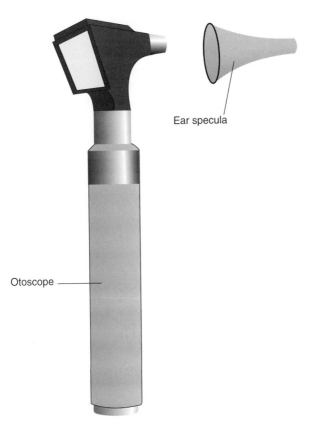

FIGURE 9-2 Otoscope.

Procedures, Techniques, and Findings

1. **Inspect the external ear**

   Note placement, size, shape, symmetry and skin color

   Observe for drainage, swelling, lumps and skin lesions

2. **Palpate the external ear**

   Feel for nodules or other irregularities

Move the pinna up and down, push on the tragus, and press behind the ear

3. **Inspect the external auditory meatus**

   Note the size of the opening, and look for any redness, swelling, discharge, or foreign body

4. **Examine the external auditory canal and ear drum with an otoscope**

   Have patient assume a sitting position

   Use largest speculum that fits comfortably in the auditory canal

   Position self to the side and slightly to the back of the ear to be examined

   Ask the patient to tip his or her head toward the shoulder opposite the ear being examined

   Using the nondominant hand grasp the pinna at the top and pull it up, back and slightly away from the head to straighten the adult ear canal; maintain this position until the otoscope is removed

   Hold the otoscope in the dominant hand in an upside-down position; brace your hand against the patient's head so that if the patient's head moves, your hand and the otoscope also move (Fig. 9–3)

   Insert the speculum into the canal (½ inch) slowly, angling it slightly downward and forward

   Avoid touching the medial wall of the canal, as it is sensitive to pain

   Observe the auditory canal for ear wax, swelling, redness, discharge, foreign bodies, lesions

   Inspect the ear drum; note color, contour, intactness

   (If the ear drum is not seen, reposition the patient's head; exert more pull on the pinna; and angle the otoscope more forward)

   Observe the position of the handle of the malleus, the umbo, the short process, and the cone of light. Rotate the otoscope as needed to visualize all areas of the ear drum (Fig. 9–4)

   Clean off any discharge or change the speculum and repeat for the other ear

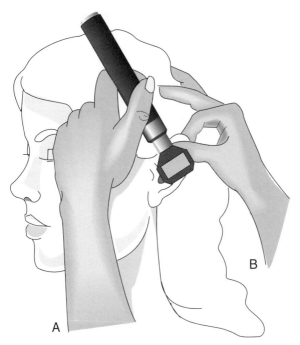

FIGURE 9-3 Method for using otoscope: *A,* Nondominant hand holds the otoscope braced against the patient's head. *B,* Dominant hand pulls the pinna up and back to straighten the external auditory canal.

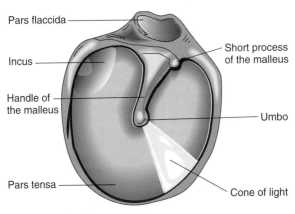

FIGURE 9-4 Ear drum.

5. Test hearing acuity (cranial nerve VIII)

Gross acuity

Position self 1 to 2 feet from patient

Voice test: Occlude one ear by placing your index finger in the external meatus and moving it back and forth gently but rapidly

Position self 1 to 2 feet from the patient

Exhale completely and with your mouth covered or the patient's eyes closed to prevent lip reading, whisper words of two equally accented syllables (baseball, arm chair) toward the ear being tested

Repeat for other ear

Lateralization of sound

Weber test: Set a tuning fork of 512 or 1024 Hz lightly vibrating by tapping the tines against your other hand (Fig. 9–5A)

Place the base of the vibrating tuning fork on top of the patient's head or in the middle of the forehead (Fig. 9–5B).

Ask the patient where the tone is heard: right ear, left ear, or both; if both, ask if loudness is equal on both sides

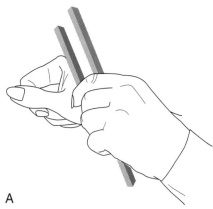

A

FIGURE 9-5 Weber test. *A,* Setting the tuning fork to lightly vibrating.

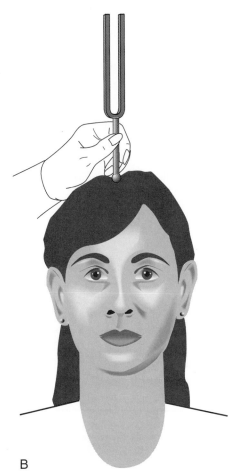

B

FIGURE 9-5 *Continued. B,* Base of the tuning fork placed on top of the patient's head.

Comparison of air and bone conduction

Rinne test: Place the base of a lightly vibrating tuning fork on the mastoid process (Fig. 9–6A)

Ask patient to say when the tone is no longer heard

When the patient no longer hears the tone quickly, move the fork so the tines are in front of the auditory meatus (Fig. 9–6B)

Ask patient if a tone is heard and direct him or her to indicate when it ends

Repeat with other ear

NORMAL FINDINGS	ABNORMAL FINDINGS

External ear

Placement

Top of pinna level with outer corner of the eye; ear angled <10 degrees toward occiput	Top of pinna below level of outer corner of the eye Unequal alignment

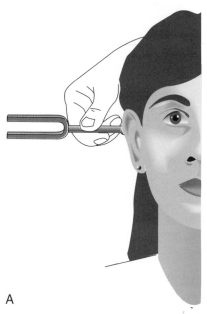

A

FIGURE 9–6 Rinne test. *A,* Vibrating tuning fork is placed on the mastoid process.

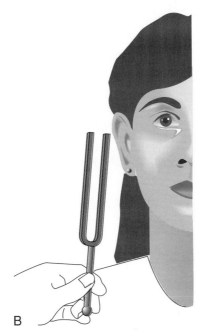

FIGURE 9-6 *Continued.* *B,* Tuning fork moved to in front of the auditory meatus.

Size
Variable but equal
(4 to 10 cm)

Excessively large or undeveloped
Unequal

General appearance
Skin intact, similar in
color to face, smooth,
uniform

Lesions, erythema, cyanosis, edema,
masses, drainage

Findings on palpation
Pinna, tragus, and
mastoid nontender on
manipulation; well-
defined bony edges
on the mastoid pro-
cess

Tenderness or pain on manipulation of pinna, tragus, or mastoid

NORMAL FINDINGS	ABNORMAL FINDINGS

External auditory meatus

Patent	Obstructed

Auditory canal

Walls pink and uniform	Marked pain on insertion of the speculum, discharge, foul odor, edema, erythema, flaking, lesions, excessive build-up of cerumen, foreign body, complete obstruction (Table 9–1)
Cilia and cerumen (wet cerumen, which is honey-colored to dark brown, or black and moist in most whites and blacks, or dry cerumen, which is gray and flaky in most Asians and Native Americans).	

Tympanic membrane

Intact, pearly gray, shiny, translucent, conical, landmarks (cone of light at 5 o'clock in right ear and 7 o'clock in left, umbo, handle of malleus, and the short process) clearly visible	Perforated or scarred, dull, blue or red, yellow-amber, retraction accentuated landmarks, bulging drum with partially occluded landmarks (Table 9–2)
Flutters when patient holds nose and swallows	No movement of tympanic membrane when patient holds the nose and swallows

Voice test (gross hearing acuity)

Able to repeat words whispered at a distance of 1 to 2 feet	Unable to hear whispered words

Weber test (lateralization of sound)

Vibratory tone heard equally in both ears	Tone lateralized to affected ear in conductive hearing loss and to unaffected ear in sensorineural hearing loss

TABLE 9-1	Variations and Abnormalities of the External Ear	
Location	Variation/Abnormality	Description and Significance
Helix	Tophi	Deposits of uric acid crystals that appear as hard, white to yellow, painless nodules
		Associated with gout, a painful metabolic bone disorder
	Darwin's tubercle	Small painless elevation typically toward top of helix
		Benign, congenital variation
	Chondrodermatitis	Small painful, indurated nodule of unknown etiology
		Most common in men
Ear canal	Otitis externa	Tender, inflamed canal
		Narrowed by swelling
	Furuncle	Infected hair follicle, which appears as a red, elevated, exquisitely tender nodule and is frequently accompanied by regional lymphadenopathy
	Polyp	Benign tumor that is red and bleeds readily
	Osteoma	Benign nontender, rock-hard, round nodule covered with apparently normal skin occurring in the inner third of the canal and obscuring the ear drum
	Exostosis	Multiple hard, round nodules of bone covered with epithelium that occur near the tympanic membrane in both ears

TABLE 9–2 Abnormal Otoscopy Findings	
Appearance of Eardrum	**Indicates**
Yellow-amber color	Serum or pus
Prominent landmarks	Retraction of drum
Air/fluid level or air bubbles	Serous fluid
Absent or distorted light reflex	Bulging of eardrum
Bright red color	Infection in middle ear
Blue or dark red color	Blood behind drum
Dark oval areas	Perforation
White dense areas	Scarring
Diminished or absent landmarks	Thickened drum
Black or white dots on drum or canal	Colony growth

NORMAL FINDINGS	ABNORMAL FINDINGS
Rinne test (comparison of air to bone conduction)	
Air conduction twice as long as bone conduction	Air conduction equal to or shorter than bone conduction with conductive hearing loss
	Air conduction longer than bone conduction (but not twice as long) with sensorineural hearing loss

Clinical Notes

Observe for signs of hearing loss during all interactions with the patient. These include a flat, monotonous tone or very loud voice, posturing of the head to direct sound to the preferred ear, the appearance of intense concentration and straining to hear, focus on the face and lips rather than the eyes of the speaker, and frequently misunderstand directions and questions or requests to repeat them.

Check the external auditory canal of all patients who wear hearing aids for irritation from badly fitting earmolds.

Never insert a speculum if a foreign object is seen in the external canal.

Geriatric Considerations

History

Wear or have worn a hearing aid? Proper fit?

History of perforated tympanic membrane?

History of cerumen impaction?

	NORMAL FINDINGS
Ear lobes	Pendulous with linear wrinkling due to loss of elasticity
	Hair growth on helix, antihelix, and tragus of pinna
External meatus	Coarse, stiff hairs at entrance
Cerumen	Drier than usual because of apocrine gland atrophy
Tympanic membrane	Whiter, duller, and thicker than in younger adult
Hearing	Presbycusis: sensory neural hearing loss characterized by initial inability to hear high-pitched tones, difficulty distinguishing consonant sounds as opposed to vowel sounds
Auditory reaction time	Increased (i.e., takes longer "to hear" and to respond)

 Pediatric Considerations

History

Known congenital hearing loss in other family members?

History of chronic and/or recurrent otitis?

Method of cleaning the child's ears?

History of child placing foreign objects in the ear?

Language development age appropriate?

Child's response to normal conversational tones?

Caretaker's intuitive feeling about the child's hearing?

Physical Examination

EQUIPMENT

Otoscope with gradient-size speculum

Pneumatic tube (an otoscope attachment that allows air to be introduced into and removed from the ear canal for the purpose of altering pressure on the tympanic membrane and thus assessing its vibrability)

PROCEDURE

To examine the internal ear of an infant pull the pinna downward since the ear canal is directed downward. To examine the internal ear of a child pull the pinna up, out, and back since the canal is directed upward and backward.

Securely restrain children, either on the caretaker's lap or an examining table, so as to prevent head movement during examination of the internal ear.

NORMAL FINDINGS	ABNORMAL FINDINGS
Infant	
Normal placement and alignment: pinna of both ears joins head at or above an imaginary line drawn across the inner and outer canthus of each eye	Low-set ears Deviation in alignment
Preauricular skin tag	Preauricular dimple Unilateral or bilateral malformation (may indicate other defects)
Tympanic membrane mobile (moves inward when air is introduced into the canal and outward when ear air is removed via a pneumatic tube)	Tympanic membrane immobile

Sound produces:

   Birth: Acoustic blink reflex

   2 weeks: Moro (startle) reflex

   10 weeks: Cessation of movement

   3 to 4 months: Turning toward sound

Absence of normal response to sound

Child and adolescent

Selective deafness

External otitis, ("swimmer's ear"): pain upon movement of pinna

Clinical Notes

Although multiple variables affect speech development, the following milestones are assessed:

   2 months: Cooing

   4 months: Babbling, squealing

   9 months: Polysyllabic vocalizing

   1 year: Single words

   2 years: Multiple-word vocabulary; combining two words

10

Assessment of the Nose and Sinuses

HISTORY AND CURRENT STATUS QUESTIONS

Rhinorrhea? Nasal stuffiness? Sneezing?	Unilateral or bilateral, pattern of occurrence: days' duration; during cold and flu season or seasonal; intermittent or continuous; associated contacts or environments; character and amount of drainage; remedies used and their effectiveness; use of drugs that cause stuffiness such as oral contraceptives, reserpine, guanethidine and alcohol; associated symptoms such as facial pain, headache, and fever
Epistaxis?	Severity, duration, associated symptoms, recurrent, other bleeding or easy bruising, any medications taken such as aspirin or warfarin
Changes in appetite or sense of smell?	Time of onset, type of change, worsened or improved with time
Allergies?	Type, treatment and its effectiveness
URIs?	Type, frequency, duration, treatment
Use of nasal sprays?	Type, how often, for what reason
Surgery or trauma?	Type, date of occurrence, residual effects
Sinus pain?	Location, severity, duration, treatment utilized, effectiveness of treatment

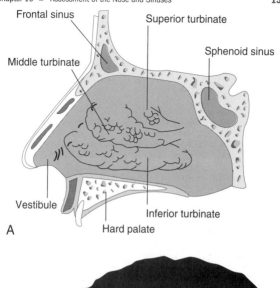

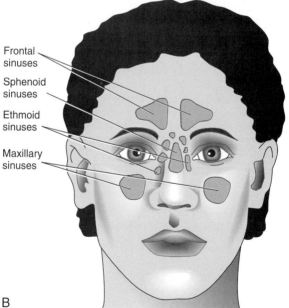

FIGURE 10-1 *A,* Anatomy of the nasal cavity. *B,* Facial sinuses (frontal view).

PHYSICAL EXAMINATION

Equipment

Otoscope with a short, wide nasal tip and a magnifying lens
   or
Nasal speculum and penlight
Small vials with familiar odors

Procedures, Techniques, and Findings

1. **Inspect the external aspect of the nose**

   Observe for asymmetry, deformity, lesions or inflammation

2. **Check patency of nares**

   Ask patient to close mouth then occlude each naris in turn

   Feel for exhaled air from the nonoccluded naris

3. **Inspect the inside of the nose**

   Mucosa

   Nasal septum

   Inferior and middle turbinates and middle meatus between them

   Use an otoscope with a short, wide nasal speculum and magnifying lens. Tilt the patient's head back and hold the handle of the otoscope to the side. Insert the speculum 1 cm into each naris in turn, taking care not to touch the septum (Fig. 10–2)

   Direct the speculum back and somewhat up to visualize both the upper and lower nose; look for color, swelling, bleeding, exudate, crusting, perforation or deviation of the septum, polyps on the turbinates, and foreign bodies

4. **Palpate the sinuses for tenderness**

   Frontal sinus

   Using pads of thumbs, press up from under the medial aspect of the brow ridges (Fig. 10–3A).

   Maxillary sinus

   Place pads of thumbs under the zygomatic arch then press up and in (Fig. 10–3B).

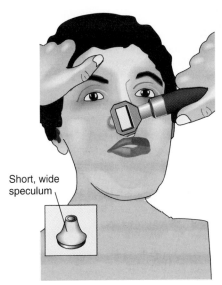

Short, wide speculum

FIGURE 10-2 Examining the naris.

5. **Test cranial nerve I**

Ask patient to close eyes; occlude one naris and hold a substance with a familiar odor beneath the other; ask the patient if anything is smelled and, if so, what it is

Repeat for other side

NORMAL FINDINGS	ABNORMAL FINDINGS
External nose	
Symmetrical	Asymmetrical; watery, purulent, mucous or bloody discharge; crusting, nasal flaring, bullous, visible vasculature, erythema
Patency of nares	
Air felt when exhaled	Noise or absence of air upon exhalation

NORMAL FINDINGS	ABNORMAL FINDINGS
Nasal mucosa	
Intact, smooth, moist pink (deeper color than oral mucosa)	Pallor, bright red or gray color, swelling, bogginess, exudate, bleeding fissures, ulcers, polyps (Fig. 10–4), tenderness

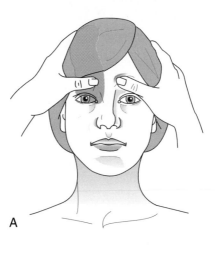

A

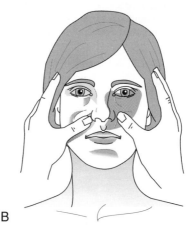

B

FIGURE 10–3 Palpating sinuses. *A,* Frontal. *B,* Maxillary.

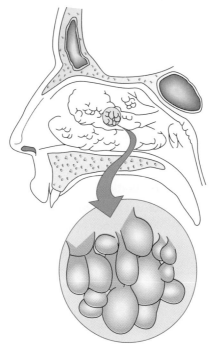

FIGURE 10-4 Nasal polyps.

Nasal septum	
Straight, uniform	Deviated
Turbinates	
Same as nasal mucosa	
Sinuses	
Nontender	Tender
Cranial nerve I	
Distinguishes odors	Unable to distinguish odors

Clinical Notes

Intranasal use of cocaine or amphetamines can cause perforation of the nasal septum. Perforation can also be due to
surgery or the long-term use of inhaled corticosteroid
therapy. Therefore, ask the patient "Have you had nasal
surgery?" and "Do you regularly take any medications?
What kind, how often do you take them, and for how long
have you taken them?"

Pale-blue tinged nasal mucosa with swollen turbinates is
characteristic of allergy; red, swollen mucosa is typical of
acute infectious rhinitis.

 Geriatric Considerations

	NORMAL FINDINGS
Nose	More prominent because of loss of subcuta-neous fat
	Coarse, stiff hairs, protruding from nostrils
Sense of smell	Decreased

Clinical Note

A decreased sense of smell may contribute to decreased food
intake and failure to detect the smell of smoke or gas.

 Pediatric Considerations

History

Mouth breathing?
Snoring?
Allergic salute?
   (See abnormal findings.)
Hyponasal phonation?
Fetid odor to breath?
Recent trauma?

Procedure

It is necessary to hold the infant's mouth closed while alternately
occluding each nostril to test for the patency of the nares.

NORMAL FINDINGS	ABNORMAL FINDINGS
Infant, child, and adolescent	
As described for the adult	Nasal flaring
	Nasal discharge
	Noisy breathing
	Encrusted, excoriated nares
	Crease across nose from frequent rubbing of the nose with the hand because of chronic nasal congestion, pruritus, sneezing, or discharge (allergic salute)

Assessment of the Mouth and Throat

11

HISTORY AND CURRENT STATUS QUESTIONS

Use of dentures?	Upper, lower, full, or partial
Dental problems (e.g., toothache, extractions)?	Type, date of onset, associated symptoms, treatment, current status
Dental examination?	Date of last examination
Bleeding gums?	Date of onset, frequency, site of bleeding, severity, presence of local lesions, tendency to bleed or bruise elsewhere
Soreness of the tongue?	Date of onset, constant or intermittent, severity, precipitating factors, local lesions, effect on eating patterns, treatment and its effectiveness
Sore throat?	
Difficulty chewing?	
Difficulty swallowing?	
Lip or oral lesions?	Type, date of onset, associated symptoms, current status
Voice changes?	Type, date of onset, duration, constant or intermittent, associated or precipitating factors

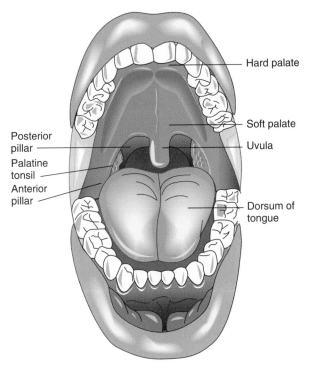

FIGURE 11-1 Major anatomical structures of the mouth and throat.

Oral surgery or injury?	Type, date of occurrence, residual effects
Oral hygiene routines?	Method (e.g., flossing, brushing, toothpaste, mouth rinse), frequency
Tobacco use?	Type (e.g., cigarettes, cigars, chewing tobacco), how much, how often, for how long (i.e., pack-years).
Alcohol use?	Type, pattern of use, amount, for how long

PHYSICAL EXAMINATION

Equipment

Light
Tongue blade
Clean gloves
Gauze square

Procedures, Techniques, and Findings

1. **Inspect the lips.**

   Observe for color, moistness, cracking, ulcers, lumps.

2. **Inspect the buccal mucosa.**

   Ask patient to remove dentures if worn. Direct patient to open mouth and then use a tongue blade and good light to observe for color, pigmentation, ulcers, nodules, or other lesions (Fig. 11–2).

3. **Inspect the gums and teeth.**

   Use tongue blade and light to observe for edema, bleeding, retraction, or discoloration of the gums. Note any missing teeth and the condition of those that remain. Have patient bite down and note alignment of upper and lower jaw.

4. **Inspect roof of mouth.**

   Use tongue blade and light to observe the color and structure of the hard palpate.

5. **Inspect all the surfaces of the tongue and the floor of the mouth.**

   Use tongue blade and light to observe tongue for discolored areas, nodules, or ulcerations. Observe dorsum of the tongue for color, surface texture, and pattern of papillae.

   Ask patient to stick the tongue out. With a gloved right hand grasp the tip of the tongue in a square of gauze and pull it left. Inspect it. Reverse procedure to inspect opposite area of tongue (Fig. 11–3).

   Observe the area under the tongue for lesions and check for tenderness.

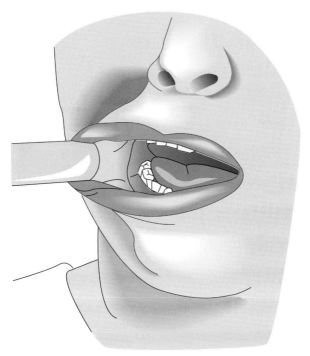

FIGURE 11-2 Use of a tongue blade to expose the buccal mucosa for examination.

6. **Inspect the structure of the throat.**

   Ask patient to open mouth. Then depress the middle of the tongue with a tongue blade. Observe for symmetry, color, exudate, ulceration, edema, and enlargement of the tonsils.

7. **Test cranial nerve X (vagus nerve, which provides motor innervation to the palate, pharynx, and larynx).**

   Use tongue blade to depress the tongue. Ask the patient to say "ah" and watch for rise of soft palate.

8. **Test cranial nerve XII (hypoglossal nerve, which provides motor innervation to the tongue).**

   Ask the patient to stick out the tongue and observe for symmetry.

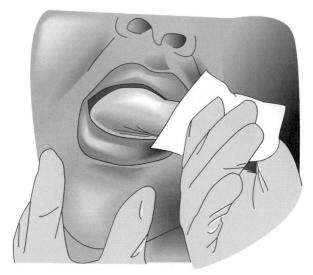

FIGURE 11-3 Grasping the tongue with a gloved hand and gauze square to inspect its sides.

NORMAL FINDINGS	ABNORMAL FINDINGS (TABLE 11-1)
Lips	
Smooth, pink, moist, intact, free of lesions	Dryness, cracks, fissures, pallor, cyanosis, drooping, involuntary movements, lesions
Blue tinge due to melanin pigment may be normal in dark-skinned persons	
Buccal mucosa	
Smooth, pink, moist, intact	Pallor, erythema, cyanosis, edema, bleeding, ulcers, white patches, other lesions
Patchy areas of hyperpig-mentation in blacks	
Gums	
Pink, moist, intact, clearly defined margins	Dryness, tenderness, edema, bleeding, ulcers, white patches, other lesions
Dark line along gingival margin may be seen in blacks	

Text continued on page 167

TABLE 11-1 Common Variations and Abnormalities of the Mouth and Throat

Location	Variation/Abnormality	Description and Significance
Lips	Herpes labialis (cold sore)	Clear vesicles that scab, often located at junction of lips and face; caused by herpes simplex virus; heal in 1-3 weeks
Gums	Hyperplasia	Enlargement of the gums that may impinge onto teeth; associated with puberty, pregnancy, and long-term use of phenytoin; also seen in leukemia
	Gingivitis	*Chronic:* red, swollen gums; may cause pain or bleed on brushing or flossing; often related to poor mouth care or poorly fitting dentures
		Acute: foul taste in mouth, malaise, occasional fever and lymphadenopathy; non-contagious infection
Buccal mucosa	Aphthous ulcer (canker sore)	Shallow pseudomembrane covered ulcer with a ring of erythema; painful; more often seen in women; cause unknown; disappears in 1-2 weeks
Buccal mucosa, tongue/lip	Leukoplakia	Areas of chalky white plaque with well-defined borders that are not easily rubbed off; associated with chronic irritation and are precancerous
Tongue	Smooth	Loss of papillae results in a very red, slick shiny appearance; associated with deficiency of vitamin B_{12}, folic acid, niacin, riboflavin, pyridoxine, and iron; accompanied by burning and dryness; also called atrophic glossitis

Table continued on following page

163

TABLE 11-1 Common Variations and Abnormalities of the Mouth and Throat *Continued*

Location	Variation/Abnormality	Description and Significance
Pharynx	Hypertrophied tonsils	Enlarged tonsils that may reach midline when tongue is protruded; enlargement is not clinically significant
	Pharyngitis	Bright red throat with patches of white or yellow exudate; swollen uvula, sore throat, fever, and large, tender cervical nodes
	Vagal nerve paralysis	Soft palate on affected side does not rise on saying "ah"; uvula deviates to nonaffected side

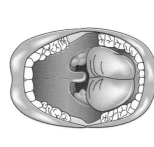

TABLE 11-1	Common Variations and Abnormalities of the Mouth and Throat *Continued*	
Location	Variation/Abnormality	Description and Significance
Chelitis	Chelitis	Inflammation with fissures, scales and crusts; painful, often chronic, and predominantly affecting bottom lip
Cheilosis	Cheilosis	Also called angular stomatitis; painful fissures in corners of mouth

Table continued on following page

165

TABLE 11-1 Common Variations and Abnormalities of the Mouth and Throat Continued

Location	Variation/Abnormality	Description and Significance
	Hairy tongue	May be black, brown, or yellow
	Geographic tongue	Red shiny areas with raised pearly borders give the appearance of a map that changes every few days; no clinical significance
	Fissured tongue	Deep irregular furrows create a scrotal appearance to the dorsum of the tongue; not clinically significant
	Varicose veins	Small, round purple or blue-black swellings on underside of tongue; appear with age and have no clinical significance

NORMAL FINDINGS	ABNORMAL FINDINGS

Teeth

| 32 pearly white and shiny, stable, smooth edges, clean and free of debris | Missing, broken, or loose teeth, cavities, dark brown discoloration |

Roof of the mouth

| *Hard palate*
Pale, moist, intact
Bony ridge down the center (torus palatinus) is a normal variation | Extreme paleness, erythema |

Frequently seen in Asians, Eskimos, and Native Americans (Fig. 11–4)

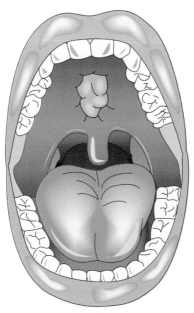

FIGURE 11-4 Torus palatinus.

NORMAL FINDINGS	ABNORMAL FINDINGS
Soft palate	
Pink, moist, intact	Erythema, pallor
Tongue	
Pink, moist, intact, smooth movement, papillae on dorsal aspect, absence of furrows	Dryness, redness, pallor, white patches, nodules, ulcers, fissures, dehydration furrows on dorsal tongue, asymmetrical contour, jerky or unilateral movement
Throat	
Mucosa pink, moist and intact; uvula midline with elevation on phonation; tonsillar pillars symmetrical	Dryness, redness, pallor, white patches, edema, ulcers or other lesions, enlarged tonsils with exudate, deviated uvula, presence of a red or gray membrane
Cranial nerve X	
Soft palate rises on "ah"	Soft palate does not rise on "ah"
Cranial nerve XII	
Symmetry of protruded tongue	Lateral deviation of protruded tongue

Clinical Notes

Third molars may be normally absent, especially among Asian and white populations.

Oral malignancies are common on the sides and bottom of the tongue.

Bright red areas of mucous membrane under dentures suggest denture sore mouth.

Palpate with a gloved finger any oral lesions to check for thickening or infiltration suggestive of malignancy.

Geriatric Considerations

	NORMAL FINDINGS
Teeth	May appear uniformly yellowed
	Receding gums with a V-shaped indentation around tooth, giving appearance of being "long in tooth"
Tongue	Smoother than in younger adult because of atrophy of papillae
	Longitudinal and latitudinal fissures may occur
Saliva	Diminished production, resulting in drier appearance of oral cavity
Buccal mucosa	Thinner and shinier than in younger adult

Clinical Note

Remove dentures during examination. Observe for fit and presence of sores or irritations secondary to friction from poorly fitting dentures.

 Pediatric Considerations

History

Does child or caretaker brush child's teeth?

Is child under the supervision of a dentist and/or orthodontist?

Fluoridated water, fluoride supplements, dose?

Drinking from a bottle or cup?

Physical Examination

PROCEDURE

When a child resists an examination of the mouth, slide a tongue blade in laterally along the buccal mucosa and insert it behind the molars to induce the gag reflex, which results in an opening of the mouth.

NORMAL FINDINGS	ABNORMAL FINDINGS
Infant	
Retention cysts on gums	Mouth breathing
Small calluses on gums and/or lips from vigorous nursing	Thrush: white plaques on oral mucosa that can not be removed
Epstein's pearls on palate	
No tonsillar tissue	
Symmetrical movement of lips, tongue, and palate with sucking	
Frenulum of tongue varies in thickness; extends to alveolar ridge	
Child and adolescent	
Large tonsils before age 10	
Symmetry of tonsils and pharyngeal pillars	
Crypts of tonsils contain concretions and/or food, which appears white	Mouth breathing
	Fetid breath
	Dental staining
	Dental caries
	Malocclusion
Geographic tongue	Smooth or cherry-red tongue
	Aphthous ulcers
	Koplik's spots

Clinical Notes

When a child presents with a croupy cough, hoarseness, throat pain, and drooling while sitting upright in order to breathe, *do not examine the oral cavity and pharynx, do not introduce a tongue blade.* These are the signs of epiglottitis, a potentially fatal condition. Examination of the oral cavity may result in complete airway obstruction.

Although there is a timetable for the sequence and eruption of primary teeth there is wide variation in normal children. Without other signs and symptoms there is no need for alarm. A general guide for children under 2 is that the child's age in months minus 6 should equal the number of teeth.

HISTORY AND CURRENT STATUS QUESTIONS

Injury?	Description, date of occurrence, symptoms, treatment, residual effects
Pain?	Date of onset; constant or intermittent; precipitating movements; associated factors (such as time of day); specific activities (such as long periods of driving, reading, or other close work)
Stiffness or limitation of movement?	Date of onset; constant or intermittent; associated factors (such as time of day); specific activities (such as long periods of driving, reading, or computer use)
Sore throat?	Date of onset, severity (e.g., ability to swallow solids, liquids, saliva), associated symptoms (e.g., cough, upper respiratory tract congestion, fever); precipitating factors

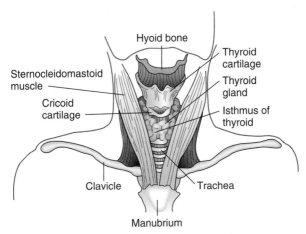

FIGURE 12-1 Anatomy of the neck.

Difficulty swallowing?	Date of onset; acute or gradual onset; constant or intermittent; ability to swallow solids, liquids, and saliva; changes in diet due to dysphagia
Hoarseness?	Acute or chronic; date of onset; constant or intermittent; precipitating factors such as overuse of voice, allergy, smoking, or exposure to other inhaled irritants; associated symptoms (e.g., cough, sore throat, fever)
Lumps or swellings?	Date first noticed, size, location, tenderness, worsened or improved since onset
Thyroid disease/surgery?	Date of occurrence, type, treatment, current medications
Recent weight change?	How much, over what period of time
Change in activity tolerance?	Ask for examples
Temperature intolerance?	Heat or cold

PHYSICAL EXAMINATION
Equipment

Stethoscope

Procedures, Techniques, and Findings

1. **Inspect the neck for appearance and position.**

   Observe symmetry and posture with patient sitting up.

2. **Check neck movement: flexion, extension, lateral abduction, and rotation.**

   Direct patient to put head back, put the chin on the chest, touch the chin to each shoulder and bend the right ear to the right shoulder and the left ear to the left shoulder without raising the shoulder.

3. **Inspect the carotid artery and jugular vein.**

   Observe for jugular distention and marked carotid pulsation.

4. **Inspect and palpate the trachea for deviation from the midline position.**

   Feel for motion.

   Place your index finger along one side of the trachea. Note the space between it and the sternocleidomastoid muscle. Repeat on the other side and compare the spaces (Fig. 12–2).

5. **Inspect the neck for the thyroid gland.**

   Direct patient to lift the chin and observe for the thyroid. Ask patient to take a sip from a glass of water, lift chin, and swallow. Observe for movement of the thyroid and if seen note its contour and symmetry.

6. **Palpate the thyroid for size, shape, and consistency.**

   Stand behind the patient and ask the patient to put the head back slightly. Place fingers of both hands on the patient's neck with the index fingers just below the cricoid cartilage (Fig. 12–3). Ask the patient to swallow and feel for the rise of the thyroid isthmus under your fingers. Move fingers down and to the sides to feel any palpable parts of the lateral lobes.

7. **Auscultate any enlarged thyroid for vascular sounds.**

   Place bell stethoscope over lateral lobes and listen.

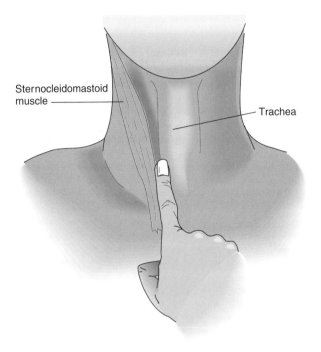

FIGURE 12-2 Palpation of the trachea for deviation.

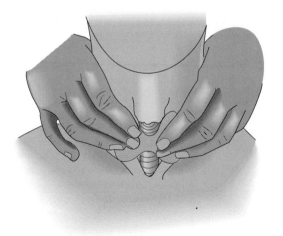

FIGURE 12-3 Position for palpation of the thyroid.

8. Palpate for cervical lymph nodes.

Using pads of first two fingers palpate both sides of the neck simultaneously. Use light to moderate pressure and move the skin over the underlying tissues rather than moving your fingers to each area. Begin in front of the ear and progress as shown in Table 12–1. To examine the submental node, palpate with one hand and place the other on top of the patient's head for support.

NORMAL FINDINGS	ABNORMAL FINDINGS
Neck	
Appearance	
Symmetrical	Unusual shortness, asymmetry, fullness, edema, masses, scars
Proportional to head and shoulders	
Movement	
From upright position:	Less than the normal range of motion
Flexion 45 degrees	
Extension 55 degrees	
Lateral abduction 40 degrees	
Rotation 70 degrees	
Coordinated, controlled movement	Uncoordinated or uncontrolled movement
Jugular vein	
	Distended
Carotid artery	
Mild pulsations	Marked pulsations
Trachea	
Midline, nontender, distinct rings	Lateral deviation, tender, edematous
Thyroid	
Usually not visible, smooth, symmetrical, and rubbery on palpation	Visible enlargement, nodular, tender, bruit

TABLE 12-1	Pattern of Palpation of Cervical Nodes
Node	**Location**
1. Preauricular	In front of ear
2. Posterior auricular	Over the mastoid process in back of the ear
3. Occipital	At the posterior base of the skull
4. Tonsillar	At the mandibular angle
5. Submaxillary	Midpoint between the mandibular angle and the tip of the mandible
6. Submental	Midline behind the tip of the mandible
7. Superficial cervical	Over the sternocleidomastoid muscle
8. Posterior cervical	Along the anterior margin of the trapezius muscle
9. Deep cervical	Deep to the sternocleidomastoid muscle
10. Supraclavicular	Deep in angle of the clavicle and sternocleidomastoid muscle

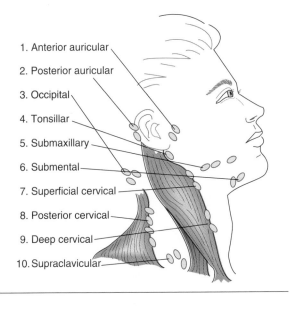

1. Anterior auricular
2. Posterior auricular
3. Occipital
4. Tonsillar
5. Submaxillary
6. Submental
7. Superficial cervical
8. Posterior cervical
9. Deep cervical
10. Supraclavicular

NORMAL FINDINGS	ABNORMAL FINDINGS
Cervical lymph nodes	
Not palpable or ≤1 cm, smooth, firm, mobile, nontender with definite margins	Palpable
	Inflamed: tender, mobile, indefinite margins
	Malignant: nontender, fixed, hard, nodular, irregular shape, indefinite margins

 Geriatric Considerations

	NORMAL FINDINGS
Submandibular salivary glands	Prolapsed and palpable as soft masses bilaterally in upper neck, below jaw
Length of neck	Shortened because of muscle atrophy and loss of fat

Clinical Note

Perform range of motion of the neck slowly, as the older patient may experience dizziness with side movements.

 Pediatric Considerations

NORMAL FINDINGS	ABNORMAL FINDINGS
Infant	
Thyroglossal duct cyst midline over trachea	Short or webbed neck indicative of genetic syndrome
Infant and child, and adolescent	
Full flexion	Nuchal rigidity: limited flexion indicative of meningeal irritation
Resistance to full flexion	Suprasternal retractions indicative of upper airway obstruction
	Torticollis: head tilted toward injured sternocleidomastoid muscle; firm mass palpated in muscle

Assessment of the Breasts and Axillae

13

HISTORY AND CURRENT STATUS QUESTIONS

Personal history of breast disease?	History of cancer, tumors, cysts, mastitis, galactorrhea, trauma, breast surgery (mastectomy, lumpectomy, biopsies, implants, or other cosmetic or reconstructive surgery), date(s) of occurrence, treatment, and outcome
Family history of breast disease?	Type of disease; age at onset; relationship of the affected person to the patient, noting maternal or paternal side as appropriate; treatment, and outcome
Breast examinations?	Frequency of breast self-examination and date last performed; frequency and date of last professional breast examination
Mammogram?	Frequency of mammograms; date and results of last mammogram
Lumps?	Location, date discovered, tender or nontender, any noticeable change in size, any relationship to menstruation
Tenderness/pain?	Localized or diffuse; unilateral or bilateral; constant or intermittent; severity; precipitating, aggravating, or relieving factors

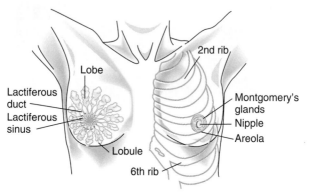

FIGURE 13-1 Anatomy of the breast.

Swelling?	Date of onset, relationship to menses, unilateral or bilateral
Skin changes?	Type, venous prominence, location, onset, sores, discolorations
Nipple discharge?	Unilateral or bilateral, color, amount, odor, frequency, associated factors and symptoms
Axillary lumps?	Location, date discovered, change in size since discovery, change related to the menstrual cycle
Axillary tenderness?	Date of onset, location, severity, precipitating and/or aggravating factors, relationship to menstruation
Axillary rash?	Date of onset, unilateral or bilateral, associated symptoms such as pruritus or burning, change in hygienic products, other potential precipitating factors

PHYSICAL EXAMINATION

Equipment

Small pillow
Sheet
Towel or gown for draping

Procedures, Techniques, and Findings

1. **Inspect the breasts for size, color, venous pattern, skin appearance, vascularity, contour, and symmetry.**

   Begin the examination with the patient in a sitting position with arms at her sides (Fig. 13–2A).

2. **Inspect the areolae for shape, color, hair, and masses.**

3. **Observe the nipples for size, shape, symmetry, and direction in which they point.**

4. **Inspect the axillae for hair distribution, cleanliness, uniformity, and skin condition.**

   Continue to inspect the breasts while the patient raises her arms over her head, lowers them, presses her hands against her hips, and, if breasts are large and pendulous, leans forward (Fig. 13–2B–D).

5. **Palpate each breast, including the tail of Spence, noting masses, consistency, tenderness, and lymph nodes.**

   With patient sitting, hands at sides, use the pads of your fingers and a firm circular motion to move the skin over the breast tissue. Proceed with palpation following a specific pattern such as spiraling out from the nipple, tracing the spokes of a wheel, or following vertical or horizontal lines (Fig. 13–3).

   Examine each quadrant and the tail of the breast. Next, repeat the palpation with the patient lying on her back with her arm (on the side being palpated) placed behind her head, and a small pillow under side to be palpated (Fig. 13–4).

   Compare the breasts to each other. If the patient reports a problem in one breast, palpate the other breast first to establish a baseline assessment, then palpate the affected breast and attempt to locate the lump or tenderness.

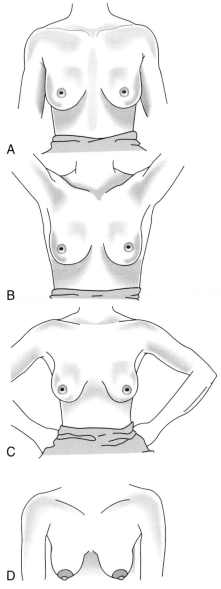

FIGURE 13-2 Positions for inspection of the breasts.

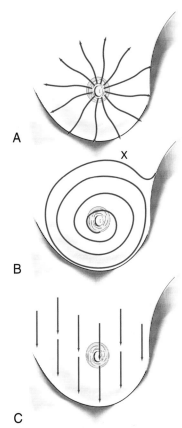

FIGURE 13-3 Patterns of breast palpation. *A*, Spokes of a wheel. *B*, Spiral.
C, Vertical lines. *Illustration continued on following page*

Verify its position with the patient when found. If a lump
is felt, describe the size, consistency, shapse, boundaries,
mobility, tenderness, and location, noting quadrant,
distance from nipple, and place on the clock (Fig. 13–5).

6. **Check for nipple discharge.**

Gently compress each nipple and note whether there is any
discharge (Fig. 13–6). Note color, consistency, quantity,

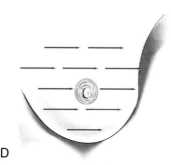

FIGURE 13-3 *Continued* *D,* Horizontal lines.

odor, presence of blood tinge or streak in *any* discharge present.

7. **Palpate the axillae.**

Ask the patient to sit and relax the arm on the side to be examined, letting it "hang down."

Use your right hand to examine the left axilla and vice versa. Use your opposite hand to support the patient's arm (Fig. 13–7).

With your fingers together and slightly cupped, reach as high into the axilla as possible.

Press inward toward the chest wall and move your fingers firmly downward to check for central nodes.

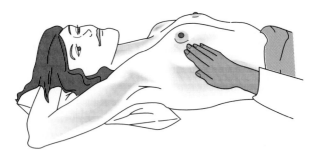

FIGURE 13-4 Recumbent position for breast palpation.

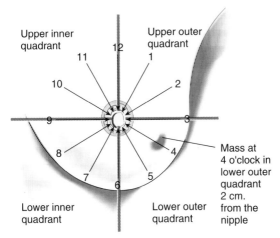

Upper inner quadrant

Upper outer quadrant

Mass at 4 o'clock in lower outer quadrant 2 cm. from the nipple

Lower inner quadrant

Lower outer quadrant

FIGURE 13-5 Noting location of a breast mass by quadrant, place on the clock, and distance from the nipple.

Repeat the maneuver, moving your fingers down the anterior border of the axilla to check for pectoral (anterior) nodes and along the inner aspect of the upper arm to check for lateral nodes.

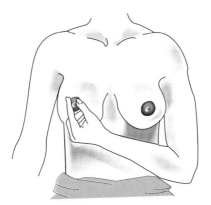

FIGURE 13-6 Nipple compression to check for discharge.

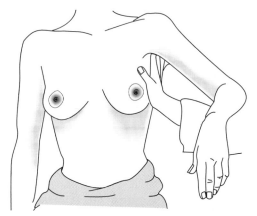

FIGURE 13–7 Position for palpation of the axilla.

Step behind the patient and repeat the maneuver, moving fingers down the posterior border of the axilla to check for posterior nodes.

Check infraclavicular nodes if enlarged or tender axillary nodes are found (Fig. 13–8).

Repeat for the opposite side.

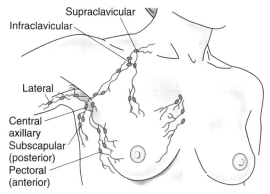

FIGURE 13–8 Location of lymph node groups draining the breast.

NORMAL FINDINGS	ABNORMAL FINDINGS
Size and symmetry	
Symmetrical, one breast may be slightly larger	Asymmetrical, marked difference in size
Contour	
Conical to pendulous	Retraction, dimpling (Fig. 13–9A), flattening, or other marked difference
Color	
Similar to normal skin on the trunk; striae often follow pregnancy.	Erythema or other discoloration
Venous pattern	
Faint, symmetrical	Asymmetrical dilation (Fig. 13–9B)
Skin appearance	
Smooth, soft	Peau d'orange (orange peel) appearance, lesions (Fig. 13–9C)
Consistency	
Uniformly loose to dense Feels firm to soft, smooth, elastic	Thickening, masses
Tenderness	
Tender if premenstrual	Tender or painful
Masses	
None	Palpable mass, feels like the tip of the nose or harder (Table 13–1)
Nipples and areolae	
No discharge Symmetrical	Discharge, retraction, deviation, recent inversion (Fig. 13–9D–E)

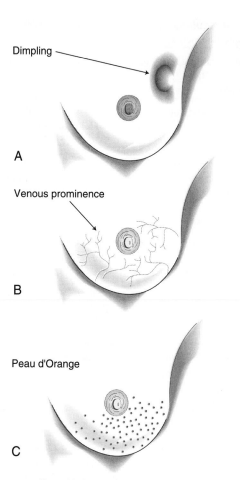

FIGURE 13-9 Observable breast abnormalities. *A,* Dimpling. *B,* Venous prominence. *C,* Peau d'orange.   *Illustration continued on following page*

Nipple deviation

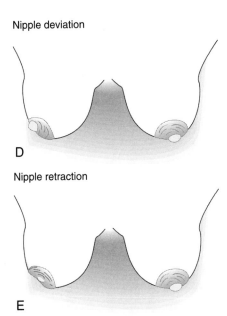

D

Nipple retraction

E

FIGURE 13-9 *Continued* D, Nipple deviation. E, Nipple retraction.

NORMAL FINDINGS	ABNORMAL FINDINGS
Axillae	
Occasionally one or more soft, nontender central nodes; otherwise not usually palpable	Palpable nodes

Clinical Notes

For men, inspect and palpate breasts in sitting position only.

TABLE 13-1 Characteristics of Benign and Malignant Breast Lumps

	Benign Cyst	Benign Fibroadenoma	Breast Cancer
Age at occurrence	30 to menopause, after which regression occurs	Puberty to 55	30 and over, with great incidence in the middle-aged and elderly
Number	Single or multiple	Usually multiple, sometimes single	Single
Shape	Round	Round, oval, or lobed	Irregular
Consistency	Soft to firm and rubbery	Usually firm	Hard
Delineation	Clearly defined edges	Clearly defined edges	Poorly defined edges
Mobility	Mobile	Mobile	Fixed
Tenderness	Often tender, especially premenstrually	Usually nontender	Usually nontender
Retraction signs			
Abnormal contour	Absent	Absent	Often present
Dimpling	Absent	Absent	Often present
Nipple retraction or deviation	Absent	Absent	Often present
Peau d 'orange skin	Absent	Absent	Often present
Increased venous prominence	Absent	Absent	Often present

Geriatric Considerations

Physical Examination

	NORMAL FINDINGS
Female breasts	Fine glandular texture due to a replacement of glandular tissue with fatty tissue
	Elongated, flat breasts as suspensory ligaments relax
Nipples	Ducts surrounding the nipple are easily palpated as firm stringy strands
	Nipples may be retracted but can be pulled out
Axillae	Sparse, gray hair

Clinical Note

Breast cancer risk increases with age. Because of the time in which they were raised, older women often find it difficult to examine their own breasts. Take time to teach breast self-examination and the need for routine mammography.

 Pediatric Considerations

History

Taking any substance including OTC medications, "herbal" or "homeopathic" remedies?

Age of thelarche (the beginning of breast development at puberty)?

Age of menarche (the appearance of the first menstrual period)?

Explore areas related to sexual precocity and sexual abuse.

Physical Examination

Note Tanner stage:

Tanner I:	No breast development
Tanner II:	Breast bud (possible asymmetry of development with tenderness)
Tanner III:	Areolae and breast tissue enlarge
Tanner IV:	Areolae and papillae form own contour
Tanner V:	Full adult maturity

NORMAL FINDINGS	ABNORMAL FINDINGS
Newborn	
Supernumerary nipples	
Leakage of milklike substance from nipples	
Infant	
Palpable breast tissue	Persistent breast tissue beyond infancy; enlarging breast buds
Adolescent	
Thelarche during preteen years	
Thelarche at 9 years	Thelarche at <8 years
Gynecomastia in males	Gynecomastia in males that does not subside with advancing maturity

Clinical Notes

Be sensitive to embarrassment and self-consciousness in the adolescent.

Assessment of the Chest and Lungs

14

HISTORY AND CURRENT STATUS QUESTIONS

Personal history of chest, pulmonary, or cardiovascular disease

History of cardiovascular disease, such as an enlarged heart, abnormal cardiac rhythm, septal or valvular defects, coronary artery disease, congestive heart failure, angina or myocardial infarction

History of pulmonary disease, such as asthma, tuberculosis, pneumonia, bronchitis, chronic obstructive pulmonary disease (COPD), sarcoidosis, or lung cancer

History of any recent or remote trauma to the chest or thorax?

History of abnormalities of or arthritic conditions involving the spine, ribs, scapula, clavicle, or sternum

Frequent muscle spasms, or at risk for occupational or recreational overuse injuries

Note age of onset, specific problem, treatment rendered (including diagnostic tests and procedures, surgery, medications, and current status)

193

Family history of chest or pulmonary disease	Any cardiovascular, pulmonary, or musculoskeletal problems affecting the thorax or lungs as described above
	Note the relation to the patient, specific problem, age of onset, age of death, and disease or problem responsible for the death of the family member
Tobacco use?	If patient or family members smoke, record type (cigarettes, cigars, pipe), how long, how many cigarettes or packs per day, for how many years (written as "pack-years")
Allergies?	Allergy to pollen, dust, other airborne irritants, medicines, drugs, food, chemicals

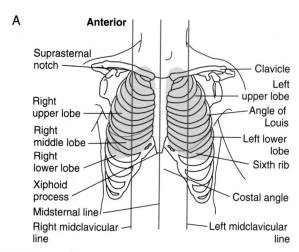

FIGURE 14–1 Thoracic landmarks. *A,* Anterior chest.

B

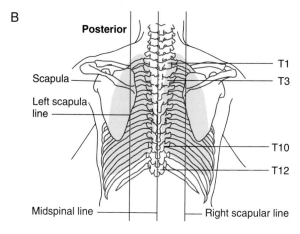

Posterior

Scapula

Left scapula line

Midspinal line

T1
T3
T10
T12

Right scapular line

C

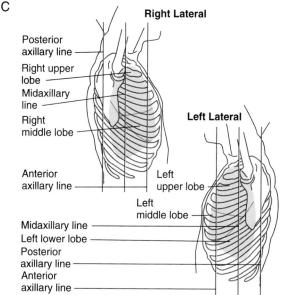

Right Lateral

Posterior axillary line

Right upper lobe

Midaxillary line

Right middle lobe

Anterior axillary line

Left Lateral

Left upper lobe

Left middle lobe

Midaxillary line
Left lower lobe
Posterior axillary line
Anterior axillary line

FIGURE 14–1 *Continued B,* Posterior chest. *C,* Right lateral and left lateral chest.

Chest pain?

Constant or intermittent, pleuritic or nonpleuritic, localized or diffuse; provocative/palliative influences, quality, region, severity and timing (PQRST) (see Chapter 1, Table 1–1).

Palpitations?

Time of occurrence (with exertion, at rest), previous ECG or Holter monitoring

Shortness of breath?

Time of occurrence (with exertion or at rest), change in respiratory rate and rhythm; evidence of a change in mental status, use of accessory muscles to breathe, cyanosis, clubbing of nails, or shift of the trachea

Cough?

Type (hacking, constant, intermittent, or rare), time of occurrence (early morning), evokes chest pain, productive or nonproductive; color and consistency of the sputum (thick, thin, clear, yellow, green, blood streaked); cultures, results

Hemoptysis?

Blood-streaked sputum or frank blood, amount (a teaspoon, a cup), duration

Associated symptoms?

Fever, chills, night sweats, nausea, vomiting, diarrhea, fatigue, malaise, weight loss, headache, dizziness, syncope, and diaphoresis

Occupational risks?

Exposure to asbestos, pollutants, chemicals, radiation, vapors and fumes

Medications?

Some medications may cause the symptoms above as side effects

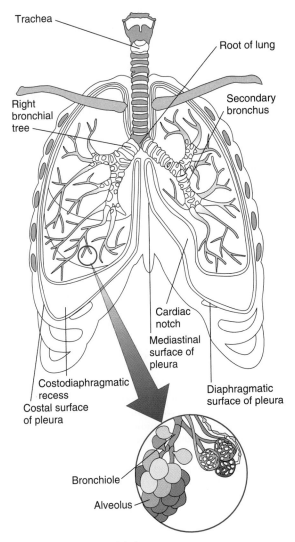

FIGURE 14-2 Anatomy of the lungs.

| Past work-up? | Chest x-ray, pulmonary function tests, arterial blood gas, lumbar sacral spine or rib film, ECG, echocardiogram, Holter monitor, exercise tolerance test, or cardiac catheterization |
| Vaccines? | Tuberculosis purified protein derivative (PPD), influenza, pneumonia |

PHYSICAL EXAMINATION

Equipment

Stethoscope

Tape measure

Procedures, Techniques, and Findings

1. **Prepare the patient for the examination.**

   Ask the patient to undress and sit up on the examining table. Observe the posterior thorax. Observe the anterior thorax with the patient lying supine.

2. **Inspect and palpate the skin and nails for color, lesions, turgor, and abnormalities.**

   Refer to Chapter 6, Assessment of the Skin, Hair, and Nails.

3. **Inspect and palpate the thorax (Figure 14–3), clavicles, scapulas, ribs, and spine for contour and abnormalities (Fig. 14–4). Note any congenital anomalies, traumatic injury, postsurgical alterations, masses, lesions, tenderness or abnormal slopes or contours.**

   Inspect as described above. Ask the patient to bend over at the waist to further inspect the curvature of the spine. Palpate and compare symmetrical areas (Fig. 14–5) of the posterior and anterior thorax using your fingertips (Fig. 14–6), or the "ball" of your hand (posterior palm).

4. **Inspect the patient's pattern of breathing; note abnormalities of rate or rhythm (Fig. 14–7).**

   Attempt to observe the patient without making him aware that you are observing his respirations. A good technique

Text continued on page 202

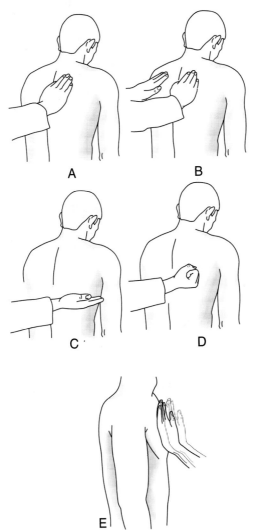

FIGURE 14-3 Thorax palpation. *A,* Use palmar surface of fingertips. *B,* Apply fingertips of both hands simultaneously. *C,* Use ulnar aspect of the hand. *D,* Use ulnar aspect of the closed fist. *E,* Place open hands simultaneously on chest.

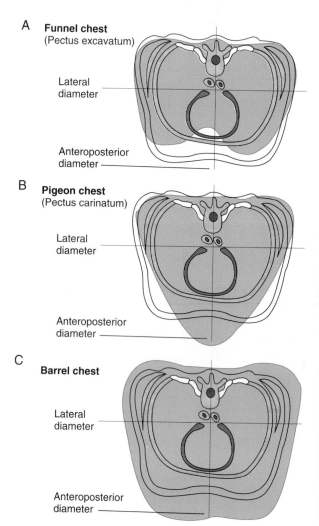

FIGURE 14-4 Abnormalities of the contour of the chest. Normal contour is indicated by solid black lines. Abnormal contour is indicated by shaded grey areas.

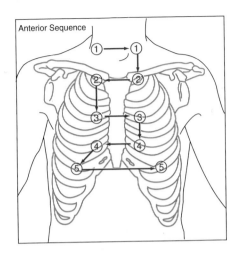

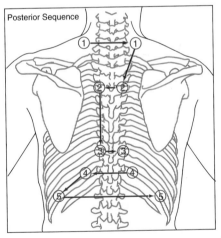

FIGURE 14-5 Compare symmetrical areas of posterior and anterior thorax.

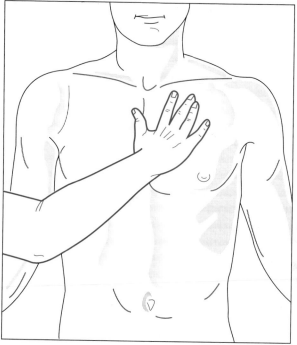

FIGURE 14-6 Palpation of the anterior thorax using fingertips.

is to pretend that you are taking the patient's pulse, while you are actually observing his respiratory pattern.

5. **Inspect and palpate the patient's breasts and axillae for shape, contour, symmetry, lesions, masses, dimpling, vasculature, and discharge.**

   Refer to Chapter 13, Assessment of the Breasts and Axillae.

6. **Palpate for tactile fremitus, the palpable transmission of sound through the chest wall.**

   Ask the patient to say "99," "99," "99" as you place the "ball" (the area of the posterior palm near the proximal finger joints) of one hand on each of the target areas as diagrammed (Fig. 14–3E). Compare the transmission of the patient's voice through the chest wall in symmetrical areas (Fig. 14–8).

7. Palpate for respiratory excursion.

Stand behind the patient with your thumbs placed on the spinal processes at the level of the tenth ribs. Spread your fingers apart over the lateral thorax [your thumbs pointing toward each other and your fingers pointing away from each other (Fig. 14–9)]. Press your palms inward toward the spine, moving your thumbs closer together with only a small skinfold between them. Now ask the patient to exhale and then take a deep breath and hold it. Observe the

Large-stem bronchi

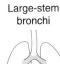

Bronchovesicular breath sounds

Lung periphery

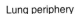

Vesicular breath sounds

Trachea

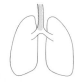

Bronchial breath sounds

A

FIGURE 14-7 *A,* Breath sounds. *I* = inspiration *E* = expiration
Illustration continued on following page

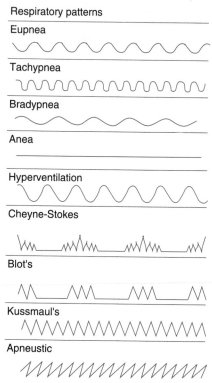

Respiratory patterns

Eupnea

Tachypnea

Bradypnea

Anea

Hyperventilation

Cheyne-Stokes

Blot's

Kussmaul's

Apneustic

B

FIGURE 14-7 *Continued B,* Respiratory patterns.

movement of your thumbs and note the expanded distance between them.

8. **Percuss the posterior and anterior thorax; the quality of the "percussion notes" will reveal the nature of underlying tissue.**

To obtain a "percussion" note, press the middle finger of your left hand firmly on the surface. Cock the middle finger of your right hand and strike the middle finger of your left hand between the distal joint and the fingernail (see Chapter 2, Fig. 2–3). Work your way down the posterior and then the anterior thorax as diagrammed

(Fig. 14–10), striking twice in each of the percussion target areas shown; listen for dullness, resonance, or tympany. Dullness will be heard over solid or fluid-filled tissue, resonance over air-filled tissue, and tympany over air-containing tissue that is hyperinflated (such as the gastric air bubble) (Fig. 14–11).

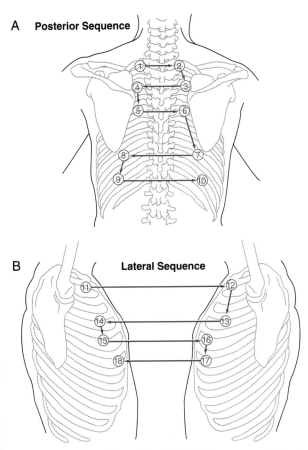

FIGURE 14-8 Palpate for tactile fremitis. *A,* Posterior sequence. *B,* Lateral sequence.   *Illustration continued on following page*

C   **Anterior Sequence**

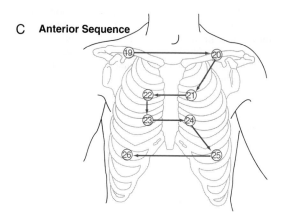

FIGURE 14-8 *Continued C,* Anterior sequence.

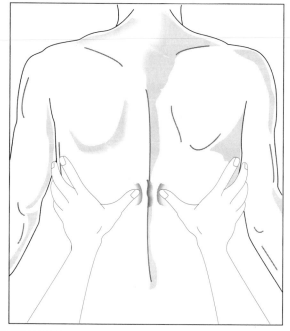

FIGURE 14-9 Palpate for respiratory excursion.

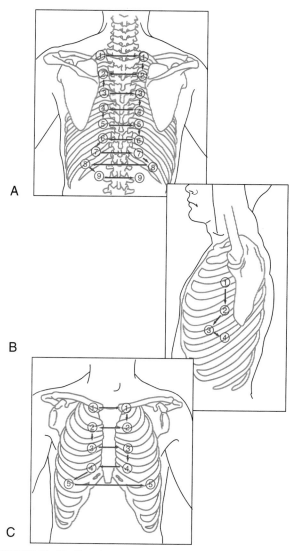

FIGURE 14-10 Thoracic percussion. *A,* Posterior sequence. *B,* Left lateral sequence. *C,* Anterior sequence.

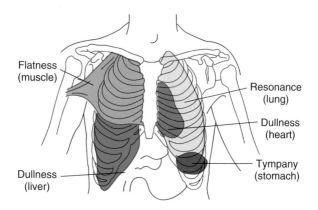

Percussion Note	Intensity	Pitch	Duration	Location Example	Disease Entity
Flatness	soft	high	short	thigh	large pleural effusion
Dullness	medium	medium	medium	liver	lobar pneumonia
Resonance	loud	low	long	lung	bronchitis
Hyper-resonance	very loud	lower	longer	none	emphysema pneumo-thorax
Tympany	loud	high	N/A	gastric air bubble	large pneumo-thorax

FIGURE 14–11 Percuss to assess the nature of underlying tissue.

9. Percuss the diaphragmatic excursion.

Ask the patient to exhale and hold it. Percuss downward from a point of resonance toward the diaphragm. Mark the point where dullness is initially heard. Ask the patient to then inhale and hold the breath. Again percuss downward from a point of resonance to the area where diaphragmatic dullness is initially heard. Mark this point and measure the distance between both points (Fig. 14–12).

10. Auscultate the posterior and then the anterior thorax in the fashion diagrammed.

Sit the patient up for both posterior and anterior chest auscultation, since abnormal findings may be masked in a supine patient. With the diaphragm of the stethoscope listen to the patient breathing. Move across and down both the posterior and then the anterior chest in the fashion diagrammed (Fig. 14–13). Discern whether artefactual sounds are occurring and eliminate them before proceeding. Further assess the rate and rhythm of the patient's breathing (see Fig. 14–7B.) Identify and distinguish vesicular, bronchovesicular, and bronchial breath sounds from artefactual and adventitious sounds (Figs. 14–14, 14–15). Note any adventitious sounds (Fig. 14–16), their timing (inspiratory or expiratory) and location, and whether they clear with coughing, deep breathing, or position changes

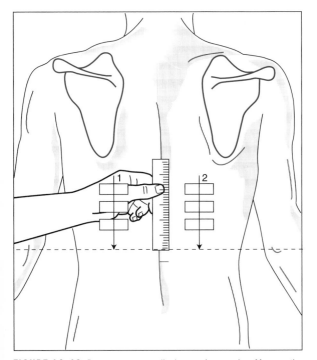

FIGURE 14-12 Percuss to assess diaphragmatic excursion. Measure the distance between the point where dullness is initially heard and where diaphragmatic dullness is initially heard.

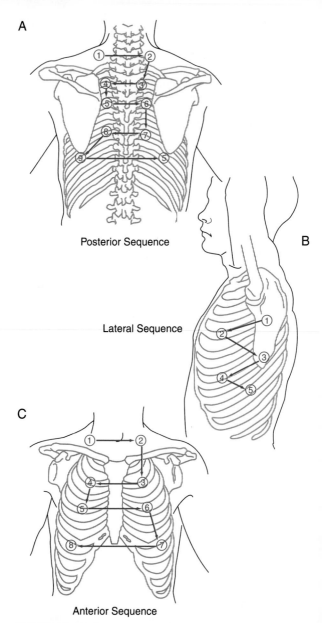

FIGURE 14-13 Auscultate the thorax. *A*, Posterior sequence. *B*, Lateral sequence. *C*, Anterior sequence.

Characteristics of Breath Sounds

Type	Duration	Intensity	Pitch	Location
Vesicular	Insp>Exp	soft	low	most of both lungs
Bronch-vesicular	Insp=Exp	medium	medium	1st and 2nd inter-spaces anteriorly and between scapula
Bronchial	Insp<Esp	loud	high	Over manubrium if heard at all
Tracheal	Insp<Exp	very loud	high	Over trachea in neck

Ratio of inspiration to expiration

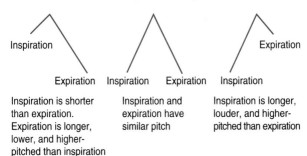

Inspiration is shorter than expiration. Expiration is longer, lower, and higher-pitched than inspiration

Inspiration and expiration have similar pitch

Inspiration is longer, louder, and higher-pitched than expiration

FIGURE 14-14 Identify breath sounds and ratio of inspiration to expiration.

NORMAL FINDINGS	ABNORMAL FINDINGS
Skin and nails	
Refer to Chapter 6	Refer to Chapter 6
Thorax	
Normal contour (ratio of anterioposterior diameter to lateral diameter equivalent to 1:2 to 5:7)	Barrel chest, funnel chest, pigeon chest, other congenital anomalies, traumatic injury, surgical alterations (see Fig. 14–4)

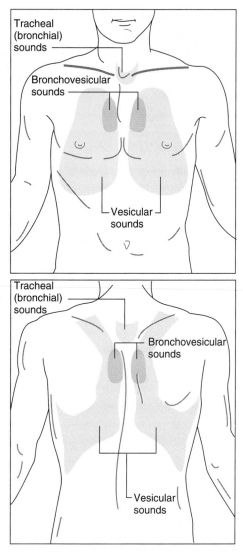

FIGURE 14-15 Distinguish vesicular, bronchovesicular, and bronchial breath sounds.

	Site auscultated	Cause	Character
Crackles (previously called rales)	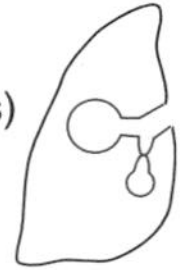 Most common in dependent lobes: right and left lung bases	Random, sudden reinflation of groups of alveoli; commonly caused by congestive heart failure, pneumonia, and atelectasis	Fine, short, interrupted crackling sounds heard during inspiration, expiration, or both; Vary in pitch: high or low; may or may not change with coughing
Gurgles (previously called rhonchi)	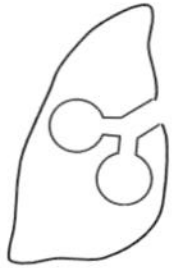 Primarily over trachea and bronchia; If loud enough, can be heard over most lung fields	Fluid or mucus in larger airways, causing turbulence	Low-pitched, continuous musical sounds heard more during expiration; May be cleared by coughing
Wheezes	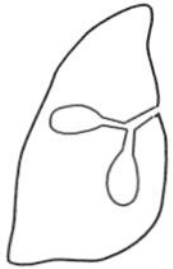 All lung fields	Severely narrowed bronchus	High-pitched, continuous musical sounds heard during inspiration or expiration; Do not clear with coughing
Pleural friction rub	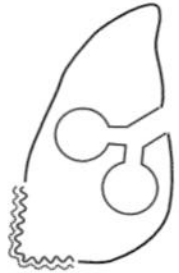 Anterior lateral lung field (if client sitting upright)	Pleura becomes inflamed; parietal pleura rubs against visceral pleura	Has grating quality; Heard best during inspiration; Does not clear with coughing

FIGURE 14-16 Adventitious sounds.

NORMAL FINDINGS	ABNORMAL FINDINGS
Ribs	
Normal sloping of the ribs	Ribs acquire more of a horizontal slope in emphysema
	Missing ribs or abnormal contour or shape secondary to surgery or trauma
Spine	
Straight, without lesions or masses	Abnormal curvatures of the spine (kyphosis, scoliosis), cysts, masses, spina bifida, or incomplete closure of the spine
Breathing	
Regular rate between 16 and 20 breaths per minute; regular rhythm in which inspiration is approximately equivalent to expiration in length	Tachypnea, bradypnea, hyperpnea, sighing, hyperventilation, ataxia, apnea, Cheyne–Stokes, Kussmaul, wheezing, whistling, respiratory lag, prolonged expiration, bulging of the intercostal spaces, use of accessory muscles
Breasts	
Refer to Chapter 13	Refer to Chapter 13
Muscles	
Normal tone, nontender	Tight spasm, tenderness, atrophy, torn or weakened (as in ventral hernia), masses
Tactile fremitus	
Should be equivalent in symmetrical areas overlying lung spaces	Decreased with a soft voice, laryngeal disease or obstruction, COPD, obstructed bronchus, effusion (fluid), fibrosis (thickening), pneumothorax (air), or infiltrating tumor; increased with increased transmission as in consolidated lung (lobar pneumonia)

Respiratory excursion

Normal respiratory excursion will separate the thumbs by 1¼ to 2 inches (see Fig. 14–9)	Limited respiratory excursion may occur with chronic fibrotic disease of the lungs, COPD, emphysema, pulmonary tumors (such as an abdominal mass), or superficial pain

Percussion

Resonance is heard over air-containing tissue and heard over most of the lung spaces; dullness is heard over fluid-filled or solid tissue and is heard normally over large underlying organs such as the liver and heart; tympany is normally heard over the gastric air bubble in the left upper quadrant (see Fig. 14–11)	Dullness replaces resonance when fluid-filled or solid tissue replaces air-containing tissue or occupies the pleural space; this occurs with pleural effusion, lobar pneumonia, abscess, blood (hemothorax), pus (empyema), and infiltration by fibrous tissue or tumor; hyperresonance is heard over hyperinflated lungs, such as in emphysema, or asthma; unilateral hyperresonance suggests pneumothorax or air-filled bulla in the lung (see Fig. 14–11)

Diaphragmatic excursion

Diaphragm descends 3 to 6 cm.	Diaphragm descends <3 cm or >6 cm

Auscultation

Artefactual sounds Normally no artefactual sounds should be heard or this will greatly confuse your results	Identify and remove all artefactual sounds such as those made inadvertently from clothing, muscle contractions, paper, scratching, examiner's fingers on stethoscope or chest

NORMAL FINDINGS	ABNORMAL FINDINGS
Breath sounds	

NORMAL FINDINGS	ABNORMAL FINDINGS
Breath sounds should normally sound symmetrical; inspiration should be approximately equivalent to expiration in duration; adventitious sounds should be absent (see Figs. 14–14, 14–15)	Longer duration of expiration is usually seen in COPD and in emphysema (see above for abnormalities in rate and rhythm of breathing)
A few individuals will normally have fine crackles present in their bilateral lung bases; otherwise, there should be no crackles, wheezes, or rubs audible	There are basically three types of adventitious breath sounds:
	Discontinuous: or coarse and fine crackles that indicate the presence of fluid in the lung spaces
	Continuous: of which there are high- and low-pitched wheezes, which indicate narrowing or partial obstruction of the airways from inflammation, mucus, edema, foreign body, or mass
	Rubs: a grating sound heard both on inspiration and expiration that is caused by the rubbing together of inflamed pleural surfaces (see Fig. 14–16)

Clinical Notes (see Fig. 14–17)

Sudden onset of chest pain and shortness of breath must be evaluated and ruled out as pain of cardiac origin or pulmonary embolus. These patients need an ECG evaluated as well as cardiac enzymes and arterial blood gas determinations. Depending on these results, further work-up may be warranted. Remember, when in doubt, it is always safest to perform the

Text continued on page 220

Condition	Auscultation	Percussion	Tactile Fremitus	Vocal Fremitus	Diaphragmatic Excursion	Trachea Position
Normal lung 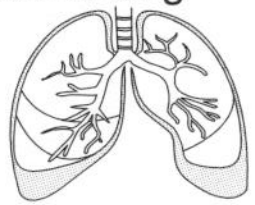	Vesicular breath sounds. No adventitous sounds	Resonant	Present and normal	Normal	3 - 5 cm	Midline
Asthma 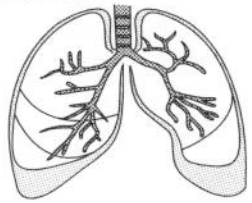	Bronchovesicular breath sounds. Wheezes or Sibilant Rhonchi are usually present.	Hyperresonant	Decreased	Decreased	Normal to slightly decreased	Midline
Atelectasis 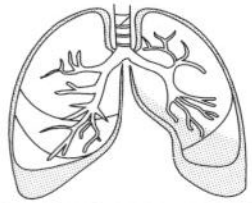	Vesicular breath sounds. Rales may be heard in late inspiration.	Dull to flat over the portion of collapsed lung. Hyperresonant over remaining unaffected portion of the lung.	Decreased or absent	Decreased or absent over affected side	Decreased on affected side	Shifted towards the affected side
Bronchitis 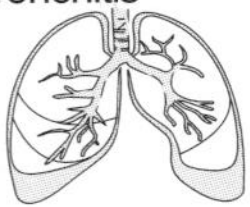	Vesicular breath sounds. Rales and Sibilant Rhonchi present.	Resonant	Normal or increased	Normal	Normal	Midline

FIGURE 14–17 Characteristics of normal versus abnormal lung conditions.

Illustration continued on following page

Condition	Auscultation	Percussion	Tactile Fremitus	Vocal Fremitus	Diaphragmatic Excursion	Trachea Position
Pneumonia and consolidation 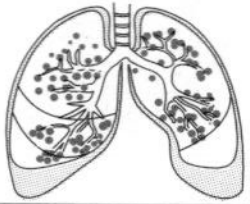	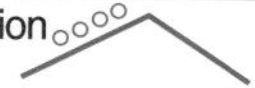 Bronchovesicular or bronchial breath sounds over the affected area. Rales may be present on late inspiration	Dull to flat	Usually increased	Usually increased bronchophony, egophony, and whispered pectoriloquy.	May be decreased on the affected side	Midline
Pneumothorax 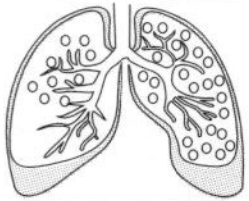	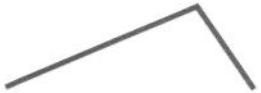 Decreased or absent breath sound. No adventitious sounds present.	Hyperresonant	Absent	Decreased or absent	Decreased on the affected side	Shifted toward the unaffected side
Pulmonary Fibrosis 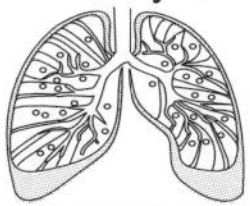	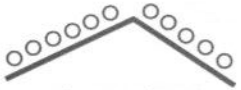 Decreased or absent bronchovesicular sounds. Rales may be heard on inspiration and expiration	Resonant to dull	Usually increased	Increased, Increased whispered pectoriloquy may be present	Decreased	Shifted toward the affected side
Tumor 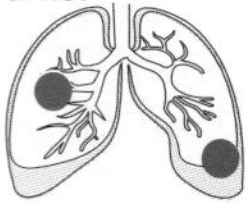	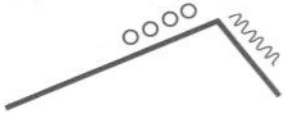 Decreased or absent breath sounds	Dull over mass	Usually increased over mass	Usually increased over mass	Decreased	May be shifted toward the unaffected side as a result of extrinsic pressure from the mass

FIGURE 14–17 *Continued* Characteristics of normal versus abnormal lung conditions.

Condition	Auscultation	Percussion	Tactile Fremitus	Vocal Fremitus	Diaphragmatic Excursion	Trachea Position
Brochiectasis 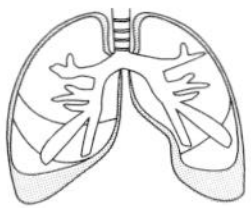	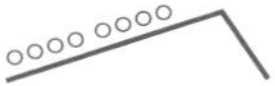 Vesicular breath sounds. Rales may be present.	Resonant or dull	Increased	Normal	Decreased on affected side.	Midline or deviated toward affected side
Emphysema 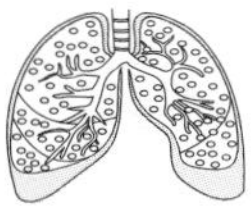	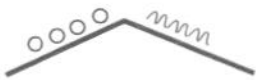 Bronchial breath sounds with prolonged expiration and decreased intensity. Fine rales are often present in late inspiration and occasional rhonchi may be heard.	Resonant to Hyperresonant	Decreased	Normal to decreased	Decreased	Midline
Pleural Effusion 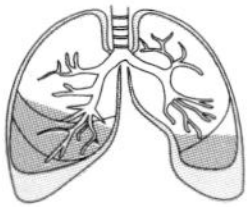	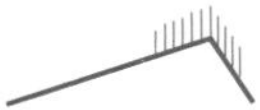 Decreased or absent breath sounds. A pleural friction rub may be heard	Dull to flat	Decreased or absent	Decreased or absent. May have brochophony, egophony, and whispered pectoriloquy if the effusion compresses the lung	Decreased on affected side.	Deviation toward the normal side

FIGURE 14–17 Continued Characteristics of normal versus abnormal lung conditions.

above minimal work-up rather than miss a potentially life-threatening diagnosis.

 ## Geriatric Considerations

NORMAL FINDINGS

Chest   Less mobile because of calcification of costal cartilages

Increased anterior-posterior (AP) diameter

Accentuation of dorsal spine, producing kyphosis

Lungs   Hyperresonance of thorax on percussion

Clinical Notes

An altered immune system, a slowed cough response, normal aging changes, and continued exposure to polluted air make the older adult more susceptible to colds, respiratory infections, and postoperative pulmonary complications. Be alert for early signs of respiratory disorders.

Provide rest times between deep breaths on auscultation to prevent dizziness and/or fainting.

 ## Pediatric Considerations

History

Mechanical ventilation as an infant?

Meconium ileus?

Has child been immunized; are immunizations up to date?

Do parents smoke?

Substance abuse: sniffing drugs (glue, cocaine, heroin)?

When the chief complaint is coughing, is the onset during the night, awaking the child from sleep, and/or with activity?

Physical Examination

PROCEDURE.   Place the stethoscope on the cheek and compare to breath sounds heard through the chest wall. This helps to differentiate referred upper airway sounds from true adventitious sounds.

Wheezes may be heard at the oral airway; crackles will *not* be heard.

NORMAL FINDINGS	ABNORMALITIES
Newborn	
Thin chest wall	
Mouth breathing	Apnea (<20 breaths per second)
Cartilaginous rib cage	
Shallow breaths	Grunting
Pectus excavatum	
Pectus carinatum	
Infant and child	
AP diameter = transverse diameter	Wheezing of bronchiolitis in infant, asthma in child
Xiphoid process protrudes anteriorly	Epiglottitis: upright posture, drooling, and air hunger
Expirations > inspirations	
Diaphragmatic breathing	
Paradoxical breathing	
Breath sounds louder and harsher than those of adults	
Hyperresonance throughout	
Diminished breath sounds are the equivalent of dullness in the adult	
Adolescent	
	Barrel chest
	Clubbing

Clinical Notes

Cough from URI persists throughout the day and may get worse upon lying flat; cough from reactive airway and/or asthma typically gets worse in the early hours of the morning and with exercise/activity.

Intensity and type of airway retractions helps localize airway obstruction:

Upper airway obstruction:	Supra/substernal retractions
Lower airway obstruction:	Intercostal retractions predominate

Decreasing "noisy" breath sounds in a child with croup may mean complete airway obstruction rather than an improvement in condition.

RAPID ASSESSMENT

THE PATIENT WITH CHEST PAIN

Ask the patient to describe the quality of the chest pain: burning, squeezing, sharp, dull, aching, crushing, stabbing, throbbing, pleuritic chest pain, pressure-like pain.

Does it feel like someone is standing on their chest?

Does the patient make the universal clenched fist sign to describe the pain?

Is the pain constant or intermittent?

Is the pain diffuse or localized?

Is the pain reproducible?

What was the patient doing when the pain occurred?

What provokes the pain and what relieves the pain?

Does the pain occur after eating?

Does the pain occur with rest or exertion?

Does the pain awake the patient at night?

Are there associated symptoms of diaphoresis, palpitations, nausea, vomiting, dizziness, shortness of breath, or syncope?

Does the patient have a fever?

Does the patient have a productive cough?

Does the patient have abdominal pain?

Change in bowel habits?

Melena or bright red blood per rectum?

Physical Examination	Rationale
Check the patient's vital signs	Rapid, slow, or irregular heart rate may indicate a life threatening arrythmia. Fever may indicate a pulmonary infection. Altered respiratory rate may indicate a pulmonary embolus.

Continued on next page

Physical Examination	Rationale
Check pulse oximetry if available	A decreased oxygen saturation indicates impaired pulmonary function
Palpate the chest and thorax	Determine whether the pain is reproducible and localized as in trauma, rib fracture, lesions, abscess, herpes zoster, or chostochondritis.
Auscultate the lungs	Abnormal breath sounds may indicate pneumothorax, effusion, infiltrate, asthma, congestive heart failure, pulmonary edema, COPD, etc.
Auscultate the heart	Check for abnormal heart sounds arrythmias, murmurs which may indicate an underlying heart disease.
Check peripheral pulses	Assess overall circulatory system. Diminished peripheral pulses may indicate occlusion or poor coronary output.
Examine the abdomen	Exclude abdominal pain mimicking chest pain (i.e. reflux esophagitis, gas pain, etc).
Examine the head, eyes, ears, nose and throat.	Determine whether the patient has upper respiratory infection.

15

Assessment of the Heart

HISTORY AND CURRENT STATUS QUESTIONS

Personal history of cardiac disease	Congenital defect, enlarged heart, arrhythmias, murmur, stenosis or insufficiency of valves, septal defects, coronary artery disease (CAD), congestive heart failure (CHF), angina, or myocardial infarction (MI)
	Hypertension (HTN), diabetes (DM), hypercholesterolemia, a history of stroke (cerebral vascular accident [CVA])
Family history of cardiac disease	Family members with any of the above-described illnesses (note: relation to the patient, specific problem, age of onset, age of death, disease/cause of relative's death)
Risk factors?	Congenital heart disease; rheumatic fever; thyroid disease; hypertension; diabetes; obesity; tobacco use; hypercholesterolemia; excessive caffeine, alcohol; or drug abuse
Chest pain?	Often patients are unable to describe the sensation they feel as "pain"; evaluate all complaints of pain with regard to the following (see Chapter 1, Table 1–1).
	Provocative factors: *What provoked the pain?*

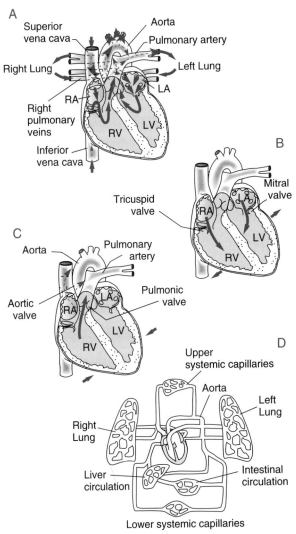

FIGURE 15-1 The cardiac cycle. *A,* Cardiac circulation. *B,* Diastole. *C,* Systole. *D,* Systemic circulation.

Exertion, rest, eating, position changes, emotions, weather changes, etc.; type and amount of activity; change in the amount of activity required to provoke the pain over time

Palliative factors: *What can the patient do to improve or alleviate the "pain"?*

Rest, nitroglycerin, position change, warmth, stress reduction

Quality: Ask the patient to describe the pain.

Patients are often unwilling to call chest pain that is cardiac in origin "pain"; they may describe discomfort, chest pressure, tightness, viselike, crushing, something heavy sitting on their chest, or make the universal sign of a clenched fist.

Region: *Where is the pain located?*

Local or diffuse; radiates to the neck, jaw, back, shoulders, or down the arms

Severity: *Is the pain mild, moderate, or severe?*

Ask the patient to rate the pain on a scale of 1 to 10 (where 10 is the most severe)

Timing: *When did the pain start?*

Occurs at a particular time of day?

Rhythm irregularities?
Are there palpitations, skipped beats, racing of the heart: when, how often; associated symptoms (shortness of breath, chest pain, or diaphoresis)?

Shortness of breath?
Does it occur unexpectedly; is it constant or intermittent; does it occur at rest or with exertion?

What type and how much activity provokes it; has this amount changed over time; occur at night, awaken patient from sleep; cause need for extra pillows; associated with cough, fever, chest pain, or diaphoresis?

Cyanosis?	Blue lips or nailbeds, ashen color of skin
Cough?	Hacking, constant, intermittent, or rare; Time of day (e.g., early morning); chest pain; productive or nonproductive: color and consistency of the sputum (thick, thin, clear, yellow, green, malodorous, blood tinged); provoked by activity, position changes, weather; alleviating factors (e.g., rest, medications)
Fatigue?	Ability to keep up with friends and colleagues; sudden or gradual onset; related to time of day
Edema?	Where and when: lower legs, ankles; at night, in the morning; pitting or non-pitting; unilateral or bilateral; any associated pain
Nocturia?	Date of onset; number of times each night; waking at night with the urgent need to urinate
Occupational risks?	Stressful occupation; exposed to smoke, pollution, toxins, vapors, fumes, strenuous exercise
Medications?	Cardiovascular medications: type, dosage, how long; side effects; any recent changes in medications or dosages
Past work-up?	Past cardiovascular tests or surgery: chest x-ray, ECG, echocardiogram, exercise stress test, Holter monitor, cardiac catheterization, angioplasty, valvuloplasty, valve replacements, or bypass Results; complications

PHYSICAL EXAMINATION
Equipment

Stethoscope
Tape measure

Procedures, Techniques, and Findings

1. **Prepare the patient for the exam.**

   Ask the patient to undress to the waist. Be sure there is adequate lighting. The patient may be examined either sitting up or supine.

2. **Inspect and palpate the anterior chest, including all six anatomical landmarks:**

   Aortic area (right 2nd intercostal space, ICS)

   Pulmonic area (left 2nd ICS)

   Erb's point (left 3rd ICS)

   Tricuspid (left 5th ICS at sternum)

   Apical (left 5th ICS at midclavicular line, MCL)

   Epigastric (just below the tip of the sternum, Fig 15–2).

   Inspect the undressed patient from the side and at an angle to take full advantage of lighting. Palpate the chest and all anatomical landmarks using the ball of the hand and posterior side of the proximal finger joints placed lightly on the chest surface in each area. Time the occurrence of any perceived pulsations, heaves (forceful pulsations that bound against the hand), or thrills (vibrations), with systole and diastole by simultaneously auscultating the heart or palpating the carotid artery.

3. **Palpate the apical impulse; this is usually the point of maximum impulse (PMI)**

   Palpate the apical area (the left 5th ICS at the MCL). You should feel a tapping sensation occurring in an area that is 1 to 2 cm in diameter and confined to one intercostal space.

4. **Palpate the carotid pulse.**

   Ask the patient to turn his/her head away from the side chosen for palpation. Observe the neck for pulsations. Place the tips of two fingers held together (usually the index and second finger) lightly over the pulsations.

   Auscultate the heart simultaneously and determine whether the carotid pulse is regular and synchronous to the first heart sound (S1).

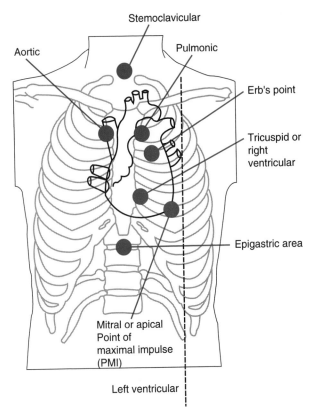

FIGURE 15-2 Location of the seven anatomical landmarks.

5. **Auscultate the heart for rate and rhythm (Fig. 15–3).**

   Using the diaphragm of the stethoscope, auscultate in the apical area of the heart (left 5th ICS at MCL) for the rate and rhythm; counting the first (S1) and second (S2) heart sounds, "lub-dub," in combination as one "beat," assess the heart rate by counting the number of beats there are in a full minute.

   Assess the cardiac rhythm. Listen to several full cycles, paying particular attention to the lengths of the systolic

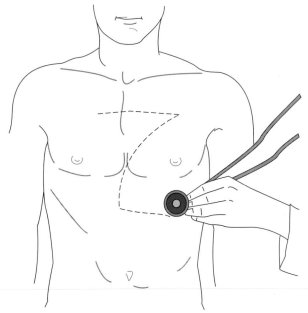

FIGURE 15-3 Auscultation of the heart for rate and rhythm.

pauses between S1 and S2, and the longer diastolic pauses between S2 and S1. Both the length of systolic and diastolic pauses should be consistent in all cycles. Any variation in length of systolic or diastolic pauses, abnormally long pauses, or sudden increase in heart rate over a number of cycles constitutes an irregular rhythm (Fig. 15–4).

6. **Compare the apical and radial pulse if the rhythm of the heart is found to be irregular.**

   Compare the apical and radial pulse by simultaneously auscultating the heart rate in the apical area while taking the patient's radial pulse. Compare the rates (beats per full minute) between the apical and radial pulse. If there is a deficit, it is usually the radial pulse that has the lower rate.

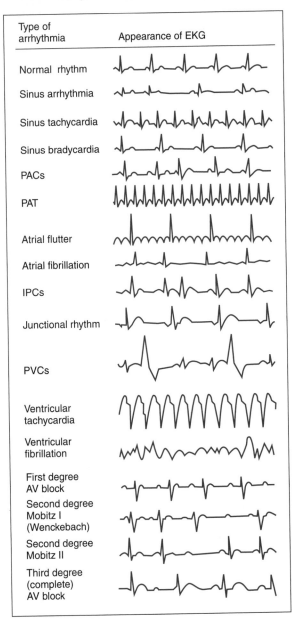

Type of arrhythmia	Appearance of EKG
Normal rhythm	
Sinus arrhythmia	
Sinus tachycardia	
Sinus bradycardia	
PACs	
PAT	
Atrial flutter	
Atrial fibrillation	
IPCs	
Junctional rhythm	
PVCs	
Ventricular tachycardia	
Ventricular fibrillation	
First degree AV block	
Second degree Mobitz I (Wenckebach)	
Second degree Mobitz II	
Third degree (complete) AV block	

FIGURE 15-4 Assessment of cardiac rhythm and irregularities.

7. **Auscultate the heart in each of the six anatomical landmarks; at each site listen for:**

   Rate and rhythm

   S1 and S2

   Systole and diastole

   Extra heart sounds

   Murmurs

   Auscultate the heart over each of the six anatomical landmarks, first with the diaphragm of the stethoscope, and then with the bell (see Fig. 15–2). Apply firm pressure when using the diaphragm, and light pressure when using the bell. It is no longer advised to limit auscultation to the landmarks alone because the sounds produced by the closing of heart valves may often be heard all over the pre-cordium; instead, edge your stethoscope across the base of the heart and down to the apex in a "Z-like" path that will include the anatomical landmarks, while at the same time covering more surface area of the heart. Listen to each heart sound carefully (Fig. 15–3).

8. **Identify and carefully auscultate the first (S1) and second (S2) heart sound.**

   The first heart sound (S1) or "lub" is followed by the shorter pause or systole. It occurs at the same time as the carotid pulse. It is heard best at the apex of the heart and is louder than the second heart sound (S2) or "dub" at the apical and tricuspid area and at Erb's point. It is softer than S2 at the pulmonic and aortic areas.

   S2 or "dub" is followed by the longer pause or diastole. It is heard best in the aortic area. It is louder than S1 at the aortic and pulmonic areas and softer than S1 in the apical and tricuspid areas and at Erb's point.

   Once you have identified S1 and S2, listen to them carefully and separately. Note whether the heart sounds are normal, accentuated (loud), or split (Fig. 15–5).

9. **Identify and auscultate systole and diastole.**

   Systole is the shorter pause between S1 and S2.

   Diastole is the longer pause between S2 and S1.

   Usually systole and diastole are silent (see Fig. 15–5).

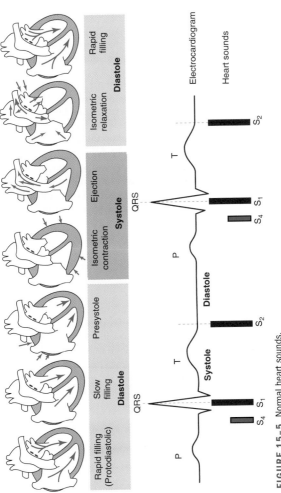

FIGURE 15-5 Normal heart sounds.

233

10. **Auscultate for extra heart sounds. Note whether there are split sounds (heard when the aortic and pulmonic or tricuspid and mitral valves do not close simultaneously), third (S3), or fourth (S4), heart sounds, or clicks audible.**

    Usually both the systolic and diastolic pauses are silent. Auscultate carefully over a number of full cycles to determine whether any extra heart sounds are occurring. You may hear a split S1 or S2, systolic clicks, prosthetic valve sounds, or an S3 or S4 (the most common sounds occurring in diastole). An S3 follows the S2 and an S4 precedes the S1. Evaluate each extra sound for location, timing, and characteristics. Be specific with descriptions of timing. State whether the sound occurs in early, mid, or late systole or diastole (see Fig. 15–6).

11. **Auscultate for heart murmurs (gurgling or blurry sounds which are produced by turbulent blood flow in the heart or great vessels). Grade the intensity of each murmur and evaluate for pattern, quality, location, radiation, and posture.**

    Murmurs occur when there is turbulent blood flow in the heart or great vessels. They are heard as a swooshing or blowing sound when auscultated. Evaluate all murmurs for intensity, pattern, pitch, quality, location, radiation, and posture.

    Intensity: The intensity of a murmur may be high, medium, or low, depending on the pressure and rate of blood flow. Grade murmurs according to the rating scale below (i.e., a moderately loud murmur would be rated III/VI):

    I: Barely audible

    II: Audible but faint

    III: Moderately loud

    IV: Loud and associated with a thrill

    V: Loud and heard with the corner of the stethoscope lifted off the chest wall

    VI: Loudest and heard easily without a stethoscope, or with a stethoscope held 1 inch above the chest wall

    Pattern: Murmurs may also vary in their intensity. They may grow gradually louder (crescendo), taper off
    Text continued on page 239

Systolic Sounds

Sound	Inspiration	Expiration	Condition
Normal heart sound	(Base) 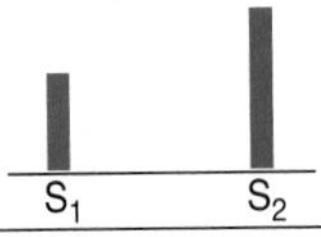 S_1 S_2	(Apex) S_1 S_2 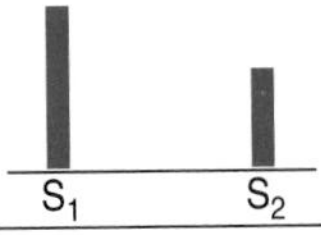	Normal heart Tetralogy of Fallot
Loud S_1	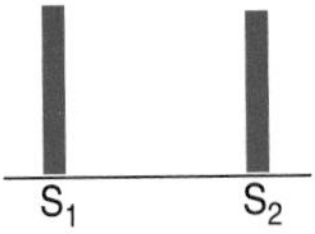 S_1 S_2		May be heard in hyperkinetic states and conditions that increase blood velocity such as exercise, fever, anemia, hyperthyroid, first degree heart block, mitral insufficiency, and severe hypertension
Varying intensity of S_1	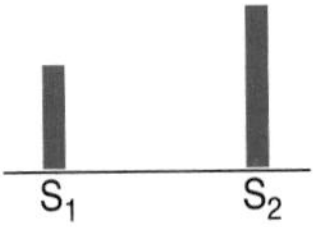 S_1 S_2	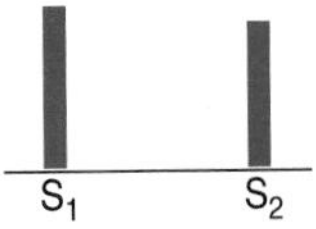 S_1 S_2	May be heard in atrial fibrillation or complete heart block with a changing systolic pause (PR interval)
Faint S_1	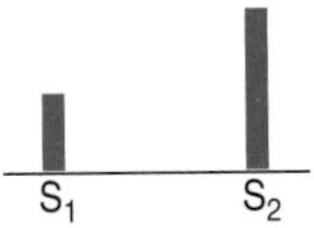 S_1 S_2	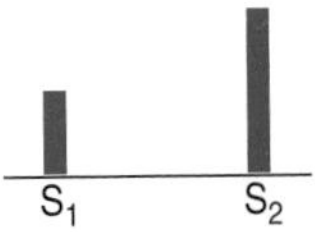 S_1 S_2	May be heard in severe hypertension, first degree heart block, and mitral insufficiency, or any condition that may increase the amount of tissue or fluid between the heart and the chest wall

FIGURE 15-6-1 Abnormal heart sounds.

Illustration continued on following page

Sound	Inspiration	Expiration	Condition
Normal splitting of S_2	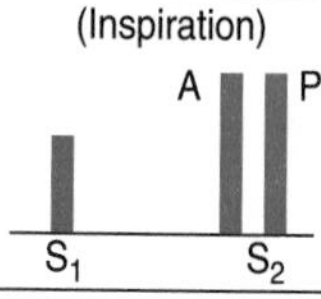 (Inspiration)	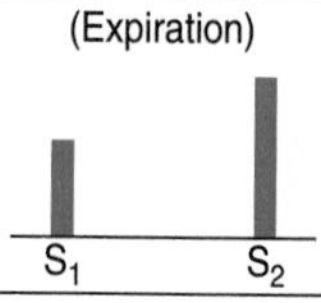 (Expiration)	Pulmonary hypertension
Wide splitting of S_2	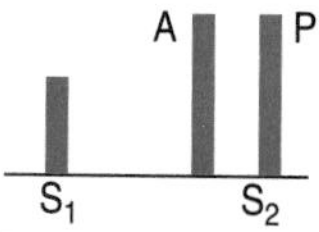	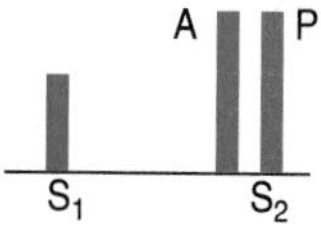	Pulmonary stenosis, mitral regurgitation, atrial septal defect, right bundle branch block
Fixed splitting of S_2	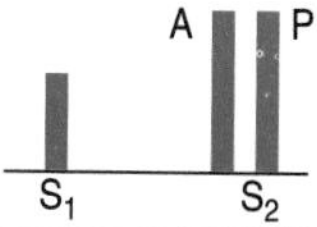	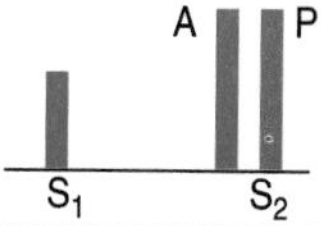	Atrial septal defect, right ventricular failure
Paradoxical splitting of S_2	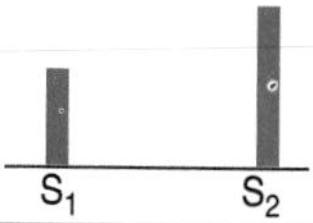	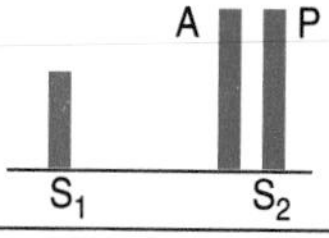	Left bundle branch block, aortic stenosis patent ductus arteriosus
Faint S_2	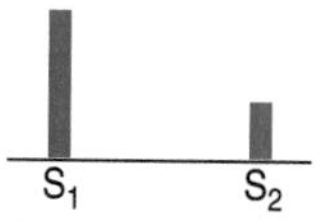	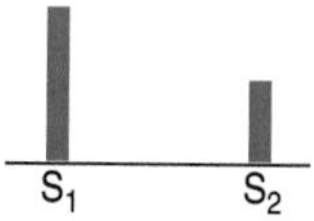	May occur with any condition that increases the amount of tissue or fluid between the heart and chest wall

Systolic Ejection Clicks

Aortic Ejection click	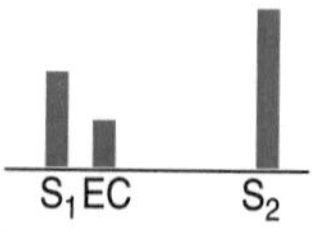	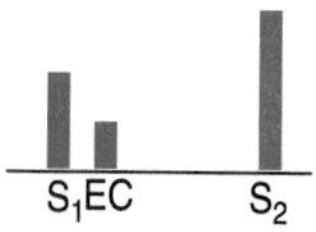	Hypertension with aortic dilation, aortic stenosis, aortic regurgitation, coarctation of the aorta, aneurysm of the ascending aorta

FIGURE 15-6-2 *Continued*

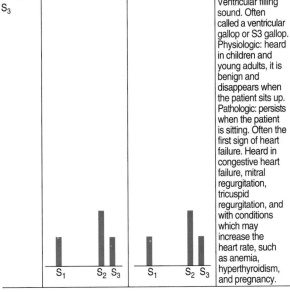

Sound	Inspiration	Expiration	Condition
Pulmonic ejection click	S_1 EC S_2	S_1 EC S_2	Pulmonic stenosis
Aortic prosthetic valve	S_1 S_2	S_1 S_2	Aortic valve replacement. Porcine valves do not produce extra prosthetic heart sounds. Prosthetic sounds are heard only with mechanical valves such as the Starr-Edwards (Ball in Cage) and the Bjork-Shiley (tilting disc) valves.

Diastolic sounds

Sound			Condition
S_3	S_1 S_2 S_3	S_1 S_2 S_3	Ventricular filling sound. Often called a ventricular gallop or S3 gallop. Physiologic: heard in children and young adults, it is benign and disappears when the patient sits up. Pathologic: persists when the patient is sitting. Often the first sign of heart failure. Heard in congestive heart failure, mitral regurgitation, tricuspid regurgitation, and with conditions which may increase the heart rate, such as anemia, hyperthyroidism, and pregnancy.

FIGURE 15-6-3 *Continued*   *Illustration continued on following page*

Sound	Inspiration	Expiration	Condition
S₄	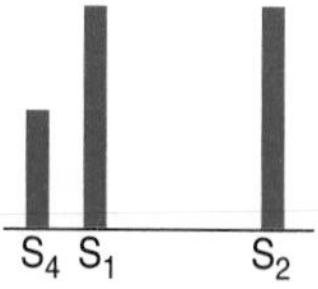 S₄ S₁ S₂	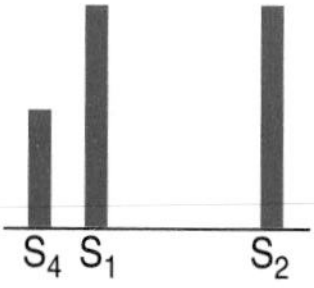 S₄ S₁ S₂	Ventricular filling sound. Often called an atrial gallop or S4 gallop. May be Physiologic: Benign. Occuring in patients over 40 years old without cardiac disease. Pathologic: Occurs with decreased compliance of the ventricle, as in cardiomyopathy, coronary artery disease, aortic stenosis, systemic hypertension, pulmonary stenosis, or pulmonary hypertension.
Opening snap of mitral valve prolapse and mitral stenosis	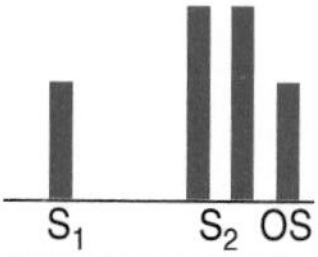 S₁ S₂ OS	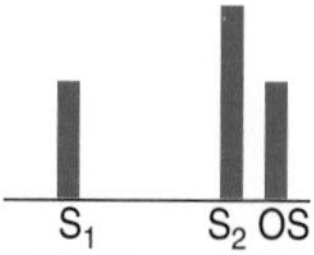 S₁ S₂ OS	Mitral valve prolapse Mitral stenosis
Prosthetic mitral valve	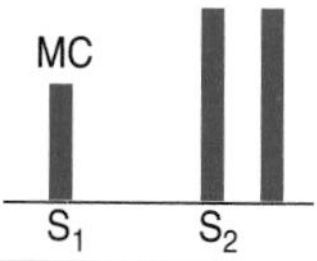 MC S₁ S₂	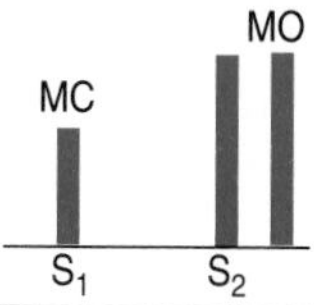 MC MO S₁ S₂	Mitral valve replacement
Opening click just after S₂	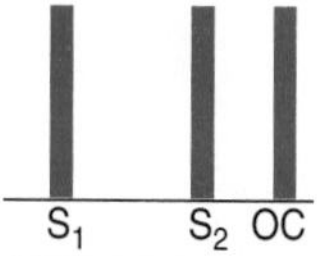 S₁ S₂ OC		May represent the opening sound of a ball-in-cage mitral valve prosthesis

FIGURE 15-6-4 *Continued*

Sound	Inspiration	Expiration	Condition
Summation sound S_3 and S_4	S_1 S_2 S_3 S_4	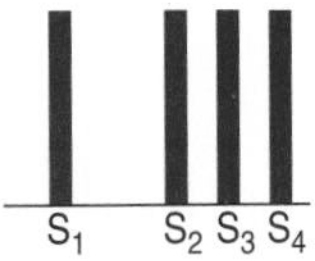	The pathologic S_3 and S_4 merge into one longer louder sound. Occurs with cardiac stress and increased heart rates.

Other variations		
Displaced apical impulses	Displaced secondary to abnormal curvatures of the spine, cardiomegaly, emphysema, obesity, increased musculature, or enlarged breasts; may be faint or barely perceivable secondary to pericardial effusions, pulmonary effusions, tumors, or any condition that may increase tissue mass or fluid between the heart and chest wall.	A small number of patients may have congenital anomalies such as dextrocardia and situs inversus, which will cause markedly abnormal findings when the borders of cardiac dullness are percussed.
Carotid bruit	Represents turbulence in the artery from atherosclerotic plaque or thrombosis	
Carotid murmur	Represents a cardiac disorder; may be transmitted to the carotid artery	

FIGURE 15-6-5 *Continued*

(decrescendo), or increase in volume to an apex and then taper off all within one systolic or diastolic pause (crescendo–decrescendo or diamond shaped).

Patterns may be pansystolic or holosystolic (or pandiastolic or holodiastolic) and occur throughout the entire length of the systolic (or diastolic) pause, or in the early, mid, or late part of systole (or diastole) (Fig 15–7).

Pitch: They may be high, medium, or low pitched.

Quality: They may be blowing, rumbling, harsh machine-like, or musical in sound.

Location: The location where murmurs are best heard may be described in terms of how many centimeters they are

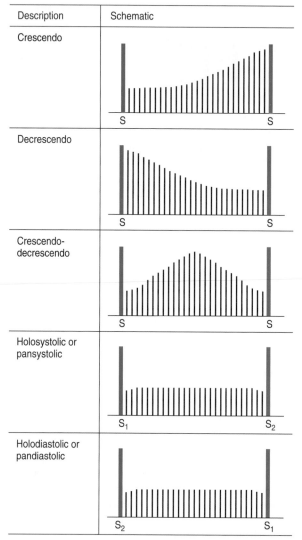

Description	Schematic
Crescendo	
Decrescendo	
Crescendo-decrescendo	
Holosystolic or pansystolic	
Holodiastolic or pandiastolic	

FIGURE 15–7 Auscultation for heart murmur intensity and pattern.

from intercostal spaces and from the sternal border, midclavicular or axillary line.

Radiation: Describe whether the murmur radiates.

Posture: Describe whether certain positions accentuate the murmur.

NORMAL FINDINGS	ABNORMAL FINDINGS
Inspection and palpation of the anterior chest	
No lesions, masses, or abnormalities; there should be a palpable pulsation, felt as a light tapping sensation, in the apical landmark at the left 5th ICS at the MCL	Any lesions, masses, or abnormalities of the chest; any palpable heaves (strong thrusting sensations) or thrills (vibratory sensations) anywhere in the precordium; any pulsations palpable in any location other than the apical landmark
Apical impulse	
The apical impulse is usually the PMI; it is confined to one ICS, in an area 1 to 2 cm in diameter	Displacement of the apical impulse or an impulse felt in an area which is larger than 2 cm in diameter
Carotid pulse	
Regular bounding rhythm that is synchronous to S1	Irregular rhythm: carotid pulse not synchronous to S1 Carotid bruit Murmur
Cardiac size	
Chest x-ray provides the most accurate assessment of cardiac size; if the percussion technique is used, the left border of cardiac dullness is usually at the 5th ICS at the MCL; the right side is on the sternal border	Increased cardiac size

NORMAL FINDINGS	**ABNORMAL FINDINGS**

Heart rate and rhythm

The average heart rate for adults is between 60 and 100 beats/minute; The average heart- rate for children varies depending on the age; The rhythm should be regular, with systolic and diastolic pauses consistent in length

Sinus bradycardia: may be normal in well-conditioned athletes

Sinus tachycardia: may occur normally after exercise

Sinus dysrhythmia: the pulse rate changes with respirations, increasing at the peak of inspiration and decreasing with expiration; occurs often in children and young adults as a normal variant

Sinus bradycardia: regular rhythm, with a decreased rate (<60 beats/minute); this may be normal in well-conditioned athletes

Sinus tachycardia: regular rhythm with an increased heart rate (>100 beats/minute); this may be normal with increased exercise

Comparison of apical and radial pulse

Usually the apical and radial pulse will be equivalent in rate and rhythm

If a pulse deficit occurs, it is usually the radial pulse which turns out to be less than the apical pulse. Any pulse deficit should be reported to a physician for further evaluation

First heart sound (S1) (see Fig. 15–6)

S1 is heard at the start of the shorter systolic pause; louder than S2 in the apical and tricuspid area and at Erb's point; softer than S2 in the pulmonic and aortic areas; normally synchronous to the carotid pulse; may be normally split (though this is rare) when the closing of the mitral and tricuspid valves are not synchronous

Loud S1

Faint S1

Varying intensity of S1

Second heart sound (S2) (see Fig. 15–6)

S2 is heard at the start of the longer diastolic pause; louder than S1 in the pulmonic and aortic areas and is softer than S1 in the apical and tricuspid areas and at Erb's point; may be normally split at the end of inspiration and return to synchronous closure (a single S2 sound) on expiration in some individuals

Fixed split S2: an S2 with a fixed split, or a split that is unaffected by respirations

Paradoxically split S2: a paradoxical split S2 will occur with expiration and disappear on inspiration

Faint S2

Systole (see Fig. 15–6)

The systolic pause is the shorter pause occurring between S1 and S2; usually silent, without extra sounds or murmurs

Early systolic sounds: Ejection clicks. An aortic ejection click is best heard at the apex and its intensity does not change with respiration. A pulmonic ejection click is best heard in the second left interspace and grows softer with inspiration

Midsystolic sounds: Midsystolic ejection clicks

Diastole (see Fig. 15–6)

The diastolic pause is the longer pause occurring after S2 and before the next S1

Early diastolic sounds:

Opening snap: a sharp, high-pitched snapping sound that occurs after S2 and is heard best in the third or fourth left ICS

Opening click heard just after S2

Summation sound (S3 + S4): the pathologic S3 and S4 merge into one longer louder sound that is often louder than either S1 or S2

NORMAL FINDINGS

ABNORMAL FINDINGS

Middiastolic sounds: S3 is a ventricular filling sound that is a dull, soft, low sound; occurs after S2 but later than an opening snap; often confused with a split S2, however, it is lower pitched than the S2, does not vary with respirations, and, unlike the S2 (which is heard best at the base of the heart), is heard best with the bell of the stethoscope at the apex or left lower sternal border

Late diastolic sounds: S4 is a very soft low sound heard just before S1; ventricular filling sound heard best with the bell of the stethoscope with the patient in the left lateral recumbent position; a physiologic S4 may occur in adults over age 40 with no evidence of cardiovascular disease

Pericardial friction rub: a high-pitched scratchy sound resembling sandpaper; best heard with the diaphragm and with the patient sitting up and leaning forward and holding breath

Systolic murmurs (Fig. 15–8)

Normally none heard

Patent ductus arteriosus (PDA): produces a continuous systolic murmur often called a machinery murmur

Atrial septal defect (ASD): produces a medium-pitched, systolic ejection murmur, best heard at the second left ICS

Text continued on page 253

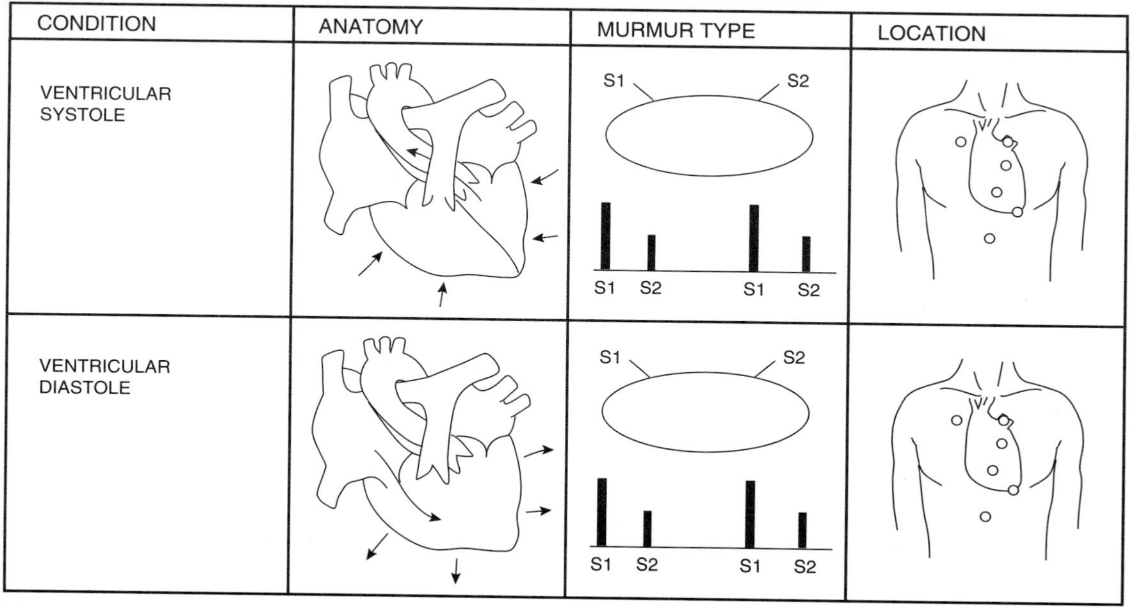

CONDITION	ANATOMY	MURMUR TYPE	LOCATION
VENTRICULAR SYSTOLE		S1 S2 S1 S2 S1 S2	
VENTRICULAR DIASTOLE		S1 S2 S1 S2 S1 S2	

FIGURE 15-8-1 Types of murmurs and their locations.

Illustration continued on following page

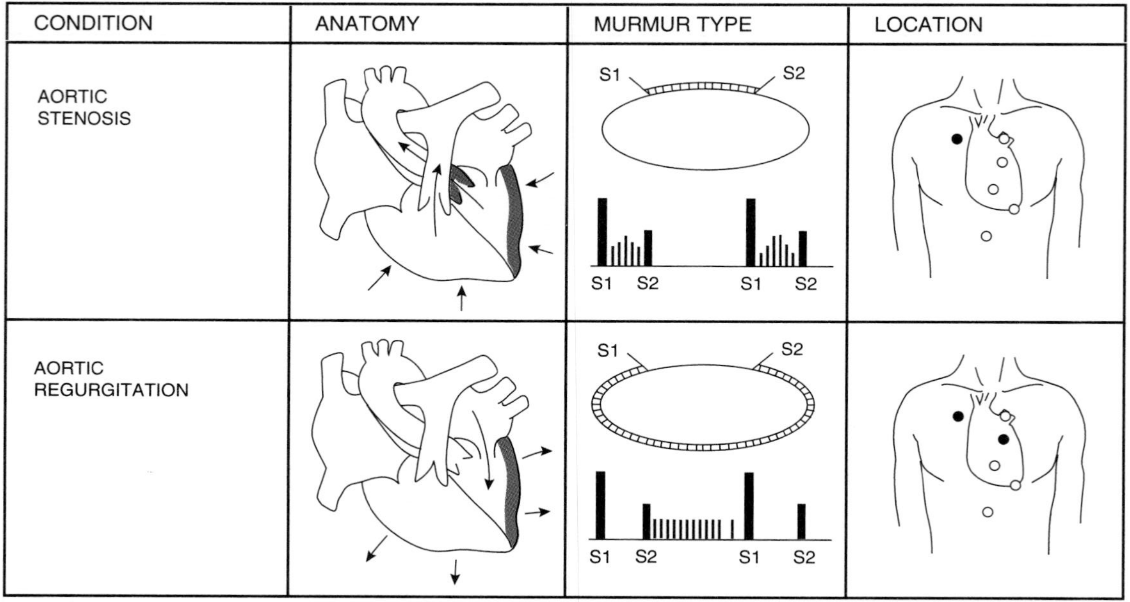
CONDITION
ANATOMY
MURMUR TYPE
LOCATION
AORTIC STENOSIS
S1
S2
S1
S2
S1
S2
AORTIC REGURGITATION
S1
S2
S1
S2
S1
S2

FIGURE 15–8–2 *Continued*

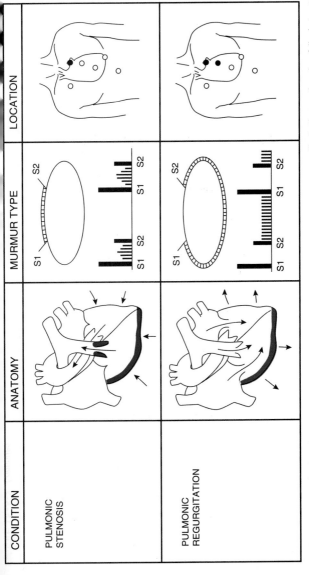

CONDITION	ANATOMY	MURMUR TYPE	LOCATION
PULMONIC STENOSIS		S1 S2 / S1 S2 S1 S2 / S1 S2	
PULMONIC REGURGITATION		S1 S2 / S1 S2 S1 S2 / S1 S2	

FIGURE 15-8-3 *Continued*

Illustration continued on following page

247

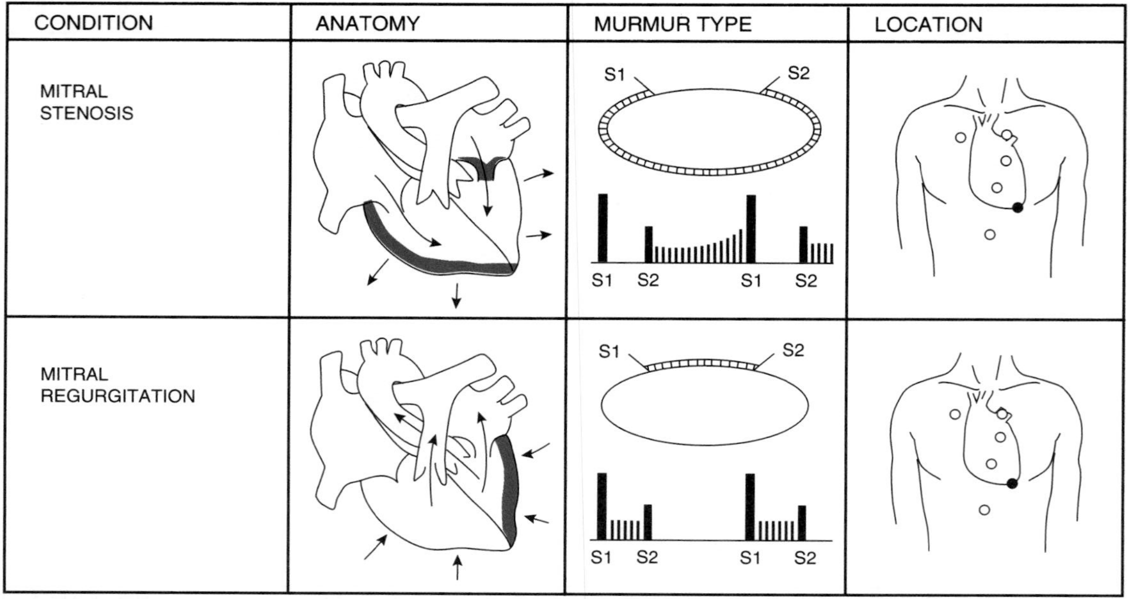

CONDITION	ANATOMY	MURMUR TYPE	LOCATION
MITRAL STENOSIS		S1 S2 / S1 S2 S1 S2	
MITRAL REGURGITATION		S2 / S1 S2 S1 S2	

FIGURE 15-8-4 *Continued*

248

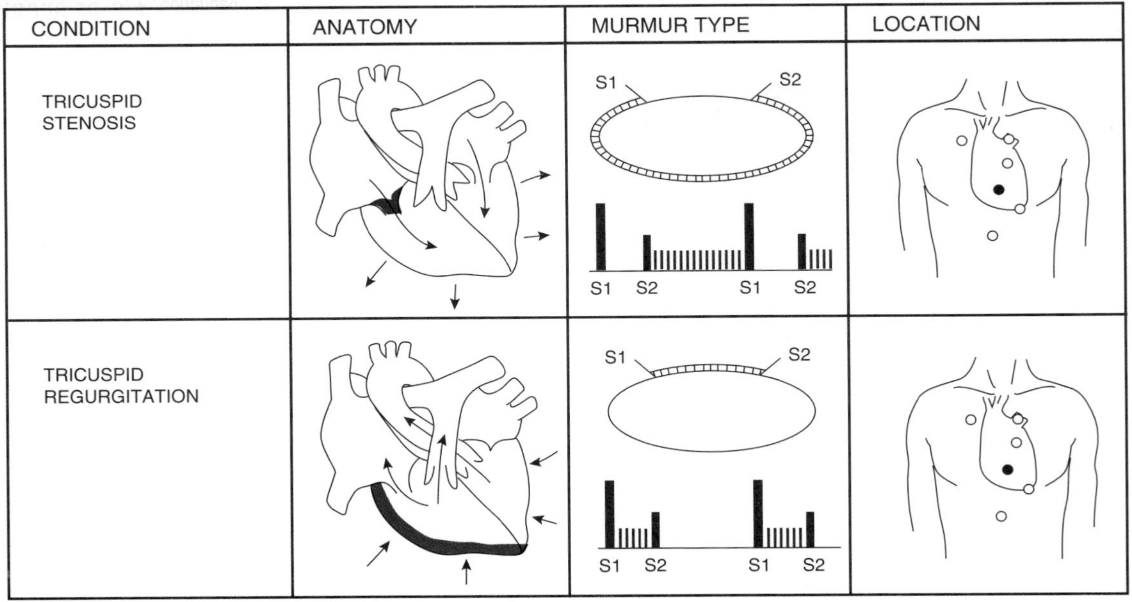
CONDITION
ANATOMY
MURMUR TYPE
LOCATION
TRICUSPID STENOSIS
S1
S2
S1 S2 S1 S2
TRICUSPID REGURGITATION
S1
S2
S1 S2 S1 S2

FIGURE 15–8–5 *Continued*

Illustration continued on following page

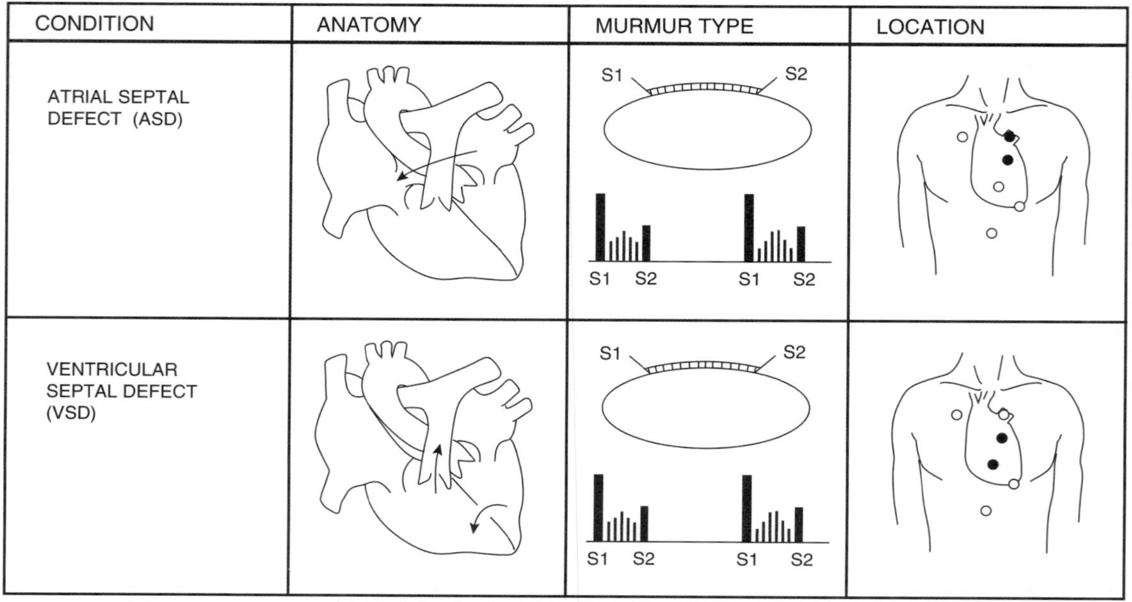
CONDITION
ANATOMY
MURMUR TYPE
LOCATION
ATRIAL SEPTAL DEFECT (ASD)
S1
S2
S1 S2 S1 S2
VENTRICULAR SEPTAL DEFECT (VSD)
S1
S2
S1 S2 S1 S2

FIGURE 15–8-6 *Continued*

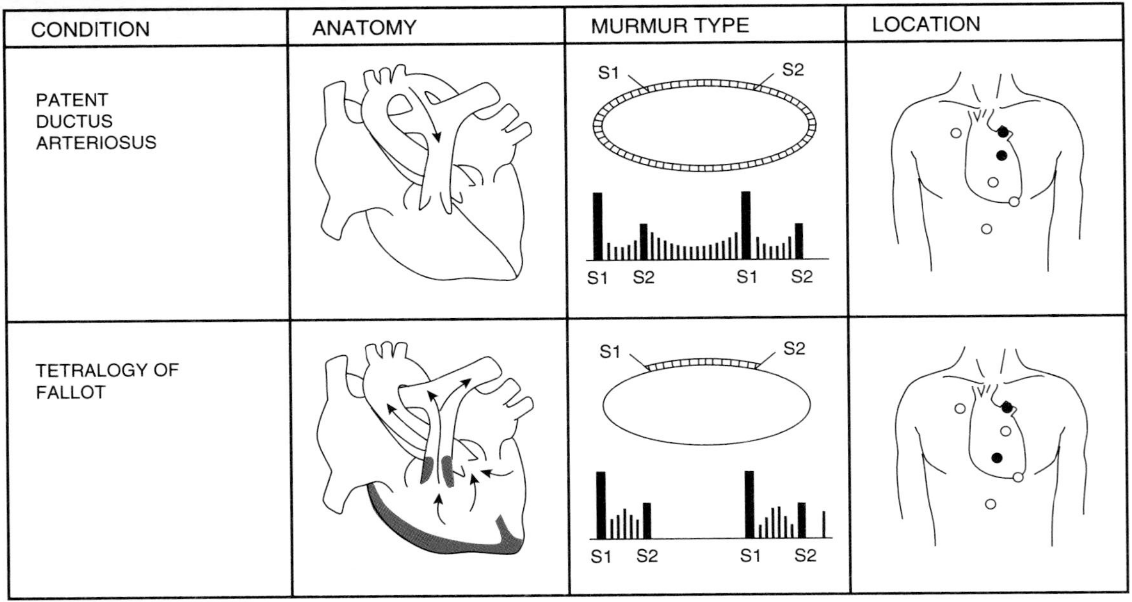

CONDITION	ANATOMY	MURMUR TYPE	LOCATION
PATENT DUCTUS ARTERIOSUS		S2 ⬭ S1 — S1 S2 S2	
TETRALOGY OF FALLOT		S2 ⬭ S1 — S1 S2 S2	

Illustration continued on following page

FIGURE 15-8-7 Continued

251

CONDITION	ANATOMY	MURMUR TYPE	LOCATION
MITRAL VALVE PROLAPSE (MVP)	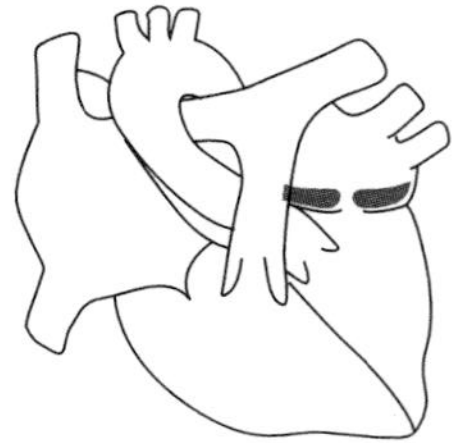	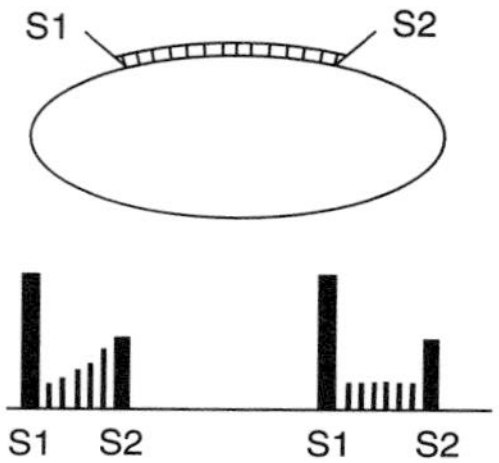	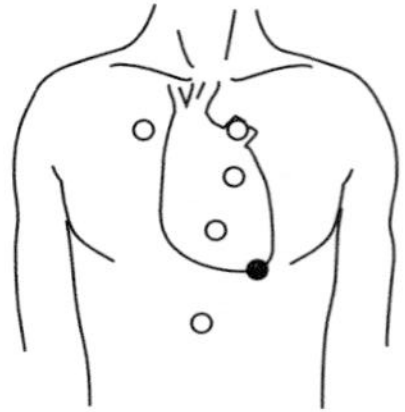
COARCTATION OF THE AORTA	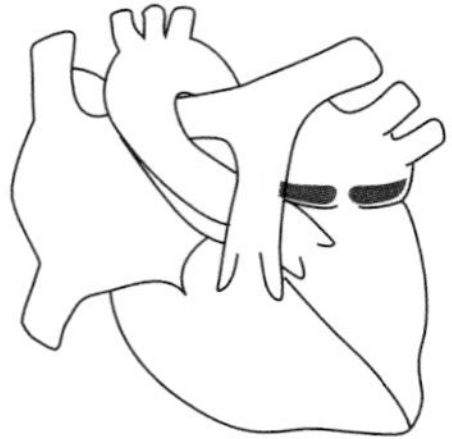	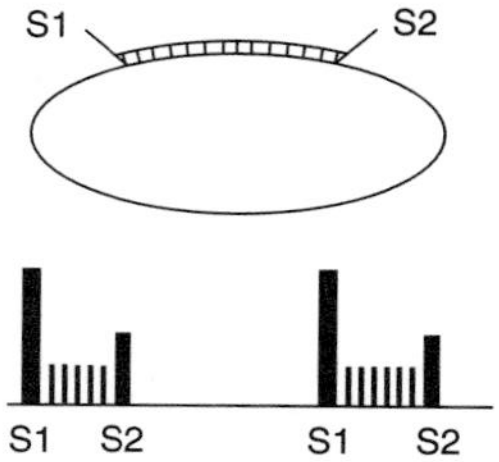	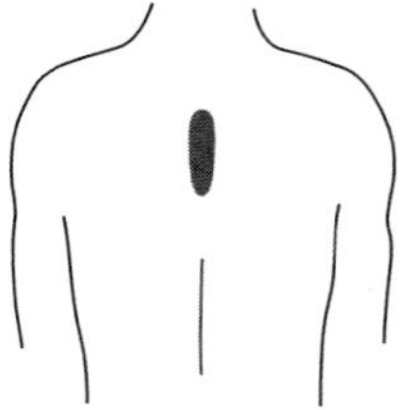

FIGURE 15-8-8 *Continued*

Ventricular septal defect (VSD): produces a loud, harsh, holosystolic murmur best heard at the left lower sternal border; in very large VSDs a soft diastolic murmur will often also be audible at the apex

Tetralogy of Fallot: produces a loud, crescendo–decrescendo, systolic murmur

Aortic stenosis: produces a loud midsystolic crescendo–decrescendo murmur, heard best at the second right ICS, which radiates to the side of the neck, left sternal border, or apex

Pulmonic stenosis: produces a medium-pitch coarse, crescendo–decrescendo murmur, best heard at the second left ICS, which often radiates to the left and the neck

Mitral regurgitation: produces a pansystolic loud, blowing, murmur, best heard at the apex, which radiates to the left axilla

Tricuspid regurgitation: produces a soft blowing, pansystolic murmur, best heard at the left lower sternal border, which increases with inspiration

Diastolic murmurs (see Fig. 15–8)

Normally none heard | Mitral stenosis: produces a low-pitched, rumbling, diastolic murmur, best heard at the apex with the patient in

NORMAL FINDINGS	ABNORMAL FINDINGS
	the left lateral recumbent position
	Tricuspid stenosis: produces a rumbling, diastolic murmur, best heard at the left lower sternal border, which grows louder with inspiration
	Aortic or pulmonic regurgitation: produces a soft, high-pitched, blowing, diastolic, decrescendo murmur, best heard at the third left ICS at the base

Clinical Notes

An ECG should be performed and evaluated to complete a thorough cardiac examination and to definitively identify arrythmias. Furthermore, an absolute diagnosis should never be made on the basis of extra heart sounds and murmurs alone. An echocardiogram or cardiac catheterization may be useful in obtaining definitive diagnoses of the causes of extra heart sounds and murmurs.

 ## Geriatric Considerations

NORMAL FINDINGS	
Rate	Longer to speed up and return to baseline in response to stress or exercise
Sound	Systolic murmurs often present because of a thickening of valves
PMI	May be displaced downward because of kyphosis

Clinical Note

Heart sounds may sound distant because of structural changes in the chest wall. To enhance the intensity of heart sounds, assist and support the patient to sit up and lean forward.

 ## Pediatric Considerations

History

Maternal therapeutic drugs during pregnancy?
Maternal substance abuse during pregnancy?

Poor feeding?

General activity level, exercise tolerance?

Squatting during play?

Circumoral cyanosis, central cyanosis versus peripheral cyanosis?

Irritability?

Physical Examination

EQUIPMENT

Newborn, infant, child, adult blood pressure cuffs

Doppler sphygmomanometer

PROCEDURE

Blood pressure must be taken on all four extremities after birth and during infancy.

Pinch nose to obliterate breath sounds for 2 seconds while evaluating the heart sounds of newborn.

NORMAL FINDINGS	ABNORMAL FINDINGS
Newborn, infant, and child	
Heart sounds: louder, high pitched, shorter duration	Unequal pulses in upper and lower extremities
	Unequal BPs in upper and lower extremities; between arms
Sinus arrhythmia	
PVCs	Gallop rhythm
Splitting of S2	
Capillary refill: 1 to 2 seconds	
	Weak suck
	Flaccid posturing
	Exercise intolerance
	Abdominal organomegaly
Peripheral cyanosis	Circumoral or central cyanosis
	Tachypnea
	Tachycardia
	Failure to thrive

NORMAL FINDINGS	**ABNORMAL FINDINGS**

Child

PMI visible, palpated at 4th ICS until 7 years old
S1 > S2 at apex

PMI:
  < 4 years: left of MCL
  4 to 6 years: at MCL
  > 7 years: right of MCL

Innocent murmur: heard in the absence of findings for cardiac disease; *systolic,* LSB, 2nd to 4th ICS, Gr. II; loudest in supine and does not radiate

Venous hum: often heard over aortic or pulmonic spaces; can be obliterated by rotating the head

Clinical Notes

Contrary to adults, pulmonary and peripheral edema are such *late* signs of cardiac failure in children that they are not considered useful indicators for diagnosis. Early signs include enlarged liver, gallop rhythm, and venous engorgement. Newborn and infant breath sounds may easily be mistaken for a murmur.

RAPID ASSESSMENT

THE PATIENT WITH SHORTNESS OF BREATH

What is the patient's actual respiratory rate?

What are the blood gas results? Pulse oximetry for oxygen saturation?

Is there tracheal deviation?

Respiratory stridor?

Jugular venous distention?

Is the shortness of breath persistant or intermittent?

Does it occur at night during sleep (PND – paroxysmal nocturnal dyspnea)?

Does it occur with exertion (DOE – dyspnea on exertion)?

Has there been a noticeable decrease in exercise tolerance?

How many blocks can the patient walk or how many stair steps can the patient climb before becoming short of breath?

Are there accompanying symptoms of fever, cough, hemoptysis, cyanosis, pallor, or URI symptoms?

Is there tachycardia, arrhythmias, or peripheral edema?

Does the patient have signs of poor circulation or DVT – deep vein thrombosis?

Does the patient have normal breath sounds?

Is the heartrate regular?

Are there audible murmurs?

Physical Examination	Rationale
Take patient's vital signs	Note tachypnea, tachycardia, low or high blood pressure or fever
Check pulse oximetry if available for oxygen saturation	This will help determine whether patient is hypoxic and requiring emergent or urgent care, and oxygen supplementation
Check for cyanosis of lips or nailbeds	Cyanosis is a sign of hypoxia
Check skin for diaphoresis	Diaphoresis may occur with pneumonia, congestive heart failure, pulmonary edema, impending myocardial infarction, and hypoglycemia
Check conjunctiva and nailbeds for pallor	Pallor of conjunctiva and nailbeds are a sign of chronic and acute anemias, which in turn may cause shortness of breath due to decreased availability of hemoglobin to transport oxygen in the bloodstream

Continued on next page

Physical Examination	Rationale
Check neck for tracheal deviation	Tracheal deviation usually indicates the presence of a pneumothorax or pleural effusion.
Check neck for jugular venous distension (JVD)	JVD usually indicates congestive heart failure.
Check lower extremities for edema	Edema in lower extremities may be dependent or positional edema, or a sign of congestive heart failure.
Auscultate the lungs for absent or abnormal breath sounds	Absent breath sounds indicate pneumothorax or pleural effusion. Crackles indicate an infiltrate (pneumonia) or congestive heart failure. Wheezes may indicate an airway obstruction or bronchitis. Expiratory wheezes indicate bronchial asthma. Friction rubs may indicate a pleurisy.
Auscultate the heart for rate and rhythm, presence of extra heart sounds, and murmurs	Heart disease may cause pleural effusions and congestive heart failure
Assess the abdomen for distention and abnormal contours	Abdominal distention may indicate ascites from congestive heart failure, obstruction, urinary retention or the presence of a mass.
Palpate the abdomen for tenderness, masses	Determine whether there is localized tenderness or a mass present in: liver, kidney, spleen, pancreas, bladder, or genitourinary tract. The female patient may unknowingly be pregnant, or have uterine or adnexal masses causing chronic anemia and shortness of breath.
Auscultate the abdomen for abnormal bowel sounds and bruits	Decreased or hyperactive bowel sounds may indicate, obstruction, perforation, ischemic bowel, diverticulitis, etc. Bruits may indicate renal artery and or aortic or femoral artery obstruction or aneurysm.
Perform rectal exam with stool guaiac	Determine whether patient is having a GI bleed, causing acute blood loss and anemia, and subsequently shortness of breath.

Assessment of the Peripheral Vascular System

16

HISTORY AND CURRENT STATUS QUESTIONS

Personal history of cardiovascular or circulatory illness	Hypertension, coronary artery disease, atherosclerotic heart disease (ASHD), high cholesterol levels, diabetes, pulmonary embolus (PE), stroke or cerebral vascular accidents (CVA), phlebitis, deep vein thrombosis (DVT), aneurysm, varicosities, vasculitis, or systemic lupus erythematous (SLE); previous vascular procedures or surgery (type); anticoagulants (which ones, for what condition)
Family history, cardiovascular or circulatory illness	Family members with any of the conditions mentioned above (family member, relation to the patient, condition, treatment rendered)
Cyanosis?	Blue nailbeds of the fingers and toes
Edema or swelling?	Bilateral or unilateral; pitting or nonpitting; associated pain
Paresthesias?	Numbness or tingling of any of the extremities

ARTERY   VEIN

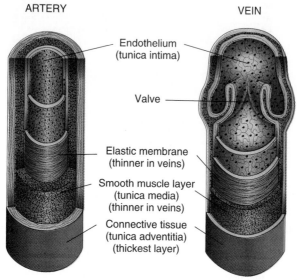

Endothelium
(tunica intima)

Valve

Elastic membrane
(thinner in veins)

Smooth muscle layer
(tunica media)
(thinner in veins)

Connective tissue
(tunica adventitia)
(thickest layer)

A

FIGURE 16-1 *A,* Arteries and veins.

Pain or leg cramps?	Time of occurrence (at night while sleeping, during the day when the patient is active); pain relief measures (massage, heat, quinine); tight stockings or garter belts worn; tendency to cross legs for extended periods of time
Temperature change?	Cold or heat intolerance or unusually cold fingers or toes (extremities equally affected, or noticeable difference in temperature between paired extremities)
Lesions and infections?	Prone to superficial infections, lesions, or ulcers on lower extremities (feet and ankles) that are slow to heal

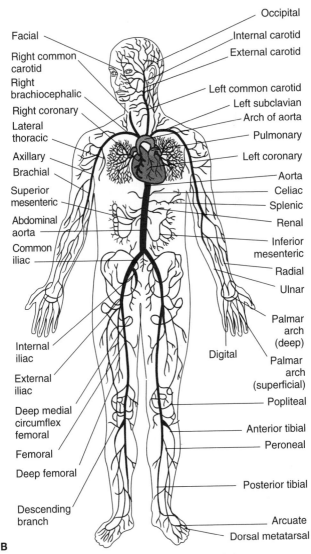

FIGURE 16-1 *Continued. B,* Systemic arterial circulation.
Illustration continued on following page

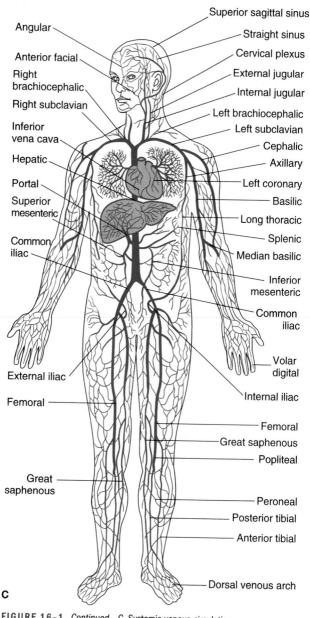

Superior sagittal sinus
Straight sinus
Cervical plexus
External jugular
Internal jugular
Left brachiocephalic
Left subclavian
Cephalic
Axillary
Left coronary
Basilic
Long thoracic
Splenic
Median basilic
Inferior mesenteric
Common iliac
Volar digital
Internal iliac
Femoral
Great saphenous
Popliteal
Peroneal
Posterior tibial
Anterior tibial
Dorsal venous arch

Angular
Anterior facial
Right brachiocephalic
Right subclavian
Inferior vena cava
Hepatic
Portal
Superior mesenteric
Common iliac
External iliac
Femoral
Great saphenous

C

FIGURE 16-1 *Continued. C,* Systemic venous circulation.

| Stasis dermatitis? | Progressively brownish discoloration of the skin (or rubor) caused by impaired circulation |
| CNS impairment? | Neurological deficits, dizziness, syncope, headaches, vision changes, change in mental status (may indicate a CVA) |

PHYSICAL EXAMINATION

Equipment

Stethoscope

Sphygmomanometer

Procedures, Techniques, and Findings

1. **Prepare the patient for the examination.**

   Ask the patient to undress to underwear and sit, stand, or lie down as necessary throughout the examination of the peripheral vascular system.

2. **Assess the patient's blood pressure (BP).**

   Using your stethoscope and sphygmomanometer, measure the patient's BP while the patient is relaxed and sitting and again just after standing. Compare BPs in each arm. Note any orthostatic changes in BP (represented by a diastolic change of >10 mmHg between sitting and standing pressures).

3. **Inspect and palpate the carotid arteries.**

   With the patient sitting, inspect and palpate the pulsations of the carotid arteries. Use the index and middle fingers together to gently palpate the carotid arteries on either side of the neck near the medial edge of the sternocleidomastoid muscle (Fig. 16–2). Examine one artery at a time. (It may help to turn the patient's head slightly away from you for inspection, and then back toward you for palpation.) Compare and note the rate, rhythm, and strength of pulsations of both carotid arteries. Note whether the rate is synchronous with the patient's heart beat and whether the rate changes with inspiration or expiration. Ask the patient to hold his/her breath, and auscultate each carotid artery for bruits using the bell of the stethoscope.

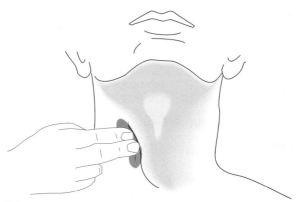

FIGURE 16-2 Palpation of the carotid pulse.

4. Assess the jugular venous pulsations.

Inspect the jugular veins with the patient sitting up at a 90 degree angle and again with the patient lying down with the head raised slightly at a 30 to 45 degree angle. Assess the level of jugular vein distention on both sides using the two-ruler method (Fig. 16–3). Note any pressures that measure > 3 cm or 1¼ inches.

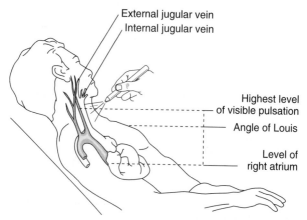

FIGURE 16-3 Inspection of the jugular vein.

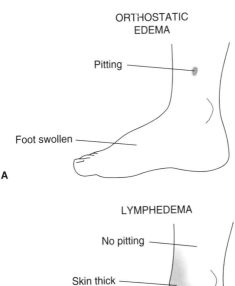

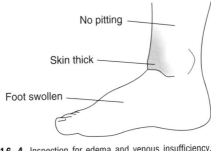

FIGURE 16-4 Inspection for edema and venous insufficiency. *A,* Orthostatic edema. *B,* Lymphedema.   *Illustration continued on following page*

5. Assess the peripheral venous circulation.

Inspect and palpate for signs of peripheral venous insufficiency (changes in the skin, changes in temperature, presence of edema, varicosities, phlebitis, and thrombosis).

Skin changes

Assess the skin, nailbeds, and extremities for signs of venous insufficiency (Fig. 16–4). Note whether there is any pallor, cyanosis, stasis dermatitis, ulcers, necrosis, edema, or cellulitis.

Temperature

Note whether the patient's fingers or toes are unusually cool to the touch. Compare paired extremities, fingers, and toes and note whether temperature changes are unilateral or bilateral.

LIPEDEMA

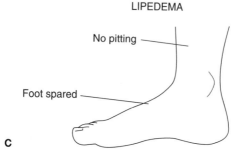

No pitting

Foot spared

C

CHRONIC VENOUS INSUFFICIENCY

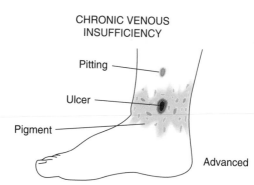

Pitting

Ulcer

Pigment

Advanced

D

FIGURE 16-4 *Continued. C,* Lipedema. *D,* Chronic venous insufficiency.

Edema

Note whether there is any edema of the lower extremities. Assess whether it is pitting or nonpitting (Fig. 16–5). Note the extent of involvement (the edema of peripheral vascular disease is usually ascending. It may begin in the ankles and ascend up the leg, depending on the severity of vascular compromise).

Varicosities

Inspect and palpate the lower extremities for varicosities. They appear as swollen, thick, tortuous veins easily seen and palpated along the surface of the lower extremities.

Phlebitis

Inspect and palpate the superficial veins for signs of phlebitis or inflammation. Look for reddened, thickened, or

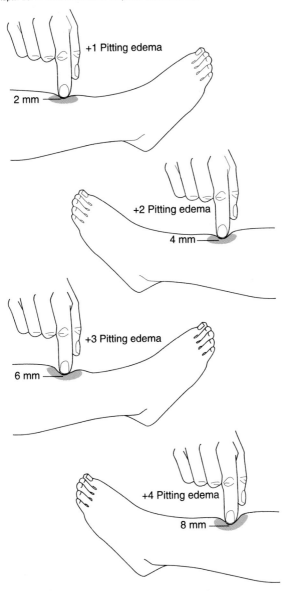

FIGURE 16-5 Inspection for pitting or nonpitting edema.

tender veins. If any occur in the lower legs, palpate the calf muscles for tenderness.

Thrombosis

Perform a special maneuver to detect DVT. With the patient's knee flexed, dorsiflex the foot. In the presence of a DVT there will be characteristic calf pain ("Homan's sign").

Special maneuvers

Phlebitis: To check for the presence of phlebitis, gently squeeze the calf muscle against the tibia and note the presence of any tenderness.

DVT: To check for DVT look for "Homan's sign." With the knee slightly flexed, dorsiflex the foot and note any occurrence of calf tenderness. The presence of calf tenderness constitutes a "positive" Homan's sign, and suggests the presence of a DVT.

Trendelenburg test: If varicosities are present, palpate the vessel with one hand while pressing down on the vessel with your second hand at a point just above the first hand. Palpate for the impulse of blood flow. Normally there should be none.

6. **Assess the peripheral arterial circulation.**

Inspect and palpate for signs of peripheral arterial insufficiency: changes in the skin and nails, changes in temperature, diminished sensation, presence of edema, pain, and diminished or absent peripheral pulses.

Skin and nails

Inspect the skin and nails. Note the presence of thin, shiny skin, scaly skin, decreased hair growth, or thickened nails.

Temperature

Note whether the extremities are cool to touch.

Sensation

Note whether the patient demonstrates any sensory deficits. Test the patient's ability to perceive soft, dull, sharp, and vibratory sensations with their eyes closed. (See Chapter 22.)

Pulses

Since each person's anatomy may vary slightly, pulses are primarily located by touch. Exert light pressure with your index and middle fingertips held together and palpate the

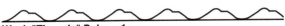

Weak "Thready" Pulse—1+
Decreased cardiac output; peripheral arterial disease;
aortic valve stenosis

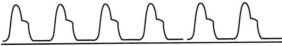

Full bounding Pulse—3+ or 4+
Hyperkinetic states (exercise, anxiety, fever), anemia,
hyperthyroidism

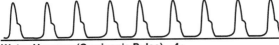

Water-Hammer (Corrigan's Pulse)—4+
Aortic valve regurgitation; patent ductus arteriosus.

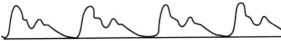

Pulsus bigeminus
Conduction disturbance, e.g., premature ventricular contraction,
premature atrial contraction.

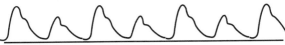

Pulsus Alternans
Left-sided congestive heart failure

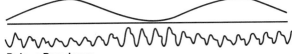

Pulsus Paradoxus
Cardiac tamponade; constrictive pericarditis

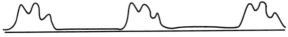

Pulsus Bisferiens
Aortic valve stenosis plus regurgitation

FIGURE 16-6 Variations in arterial pulses.

arterial pulses. Use deep palpation if needed to locate the femoral artery. Compare all contralateral or paired pulses for rhythm, strength, and equality (Fig. 16–6). If the pulse is difficult to find, or not readily palpable, you may use a doppler, or ultrasound, stethoscope to auscultate for the pulse.

Radial pulse

Palpate the radial pulse along the radial groove on the palmar and radial side of the wrist (Fig. 16–7A).

Ulnar pulse

Palpate the ulnar pulse on the palmar and medial side of the wrist (Fig. 16–7B).

Brachial pulse

Palpate the brachial pulse at the antecubital fossa between the biceps and triceps muscles (Fig. 16–7C).

Femoral pulse

With the patient supine, palpate the femoral pulse just below the inguinal ligament and halfway between the symphysis pubis and the anterior superior iliac spine (Fig. 16–7D).

Location of popliteal pulse

Palpate the popliteal pulse located behind the knee with the patient supine or prone. Ask the patient to relax the leg muscles and slightly flex the knee (Fig. 16–7E).

Location of dorsalis pedis pulse

Palpate the dorsalis pedis pulse with the patient supine. It can be found on the anterior or upper aspect of the foot, halfway between the base of the ankle and the second metatarsophalangeal joint (Fig. 16–7F).

Location of posterior tibial pulse

Palpate the posterior tibial pulse just below and behind the medial malleolus with the foot relaxed and slightly extended (Fig. 16–7G).

Special maneuvers

Allen test: If there are decreased radial or ulnar pulses in the patient's wrist perform the Allen test. Ask the patient to make a fist, then simultaneously obliterate both the ulnar and radial pulses by exerting pressure with your finger tips.

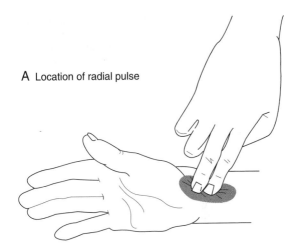

A Location of radial pulse

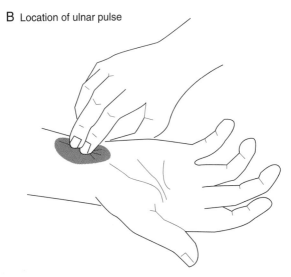

B Location of ulnar pulse

FIGURE 16-7 Location of pulses.
Illustration continued on following page

Ask the patient to open the fist and release the radial artery. Normally the full palm will become pink. If only half of the palm becomes pink, it is a sign of radial arterial insufficiency. Repeat the test, and this time release only the ulnar artery. Again assess whether there is full or half flushing of the palm. Flushing of half of the palm suggests ulnar arterial insufficiency. Lower extremities: If there are diminished pulses in the lower extremities perform two special maneuvers. First, with the patient supine, elevate the

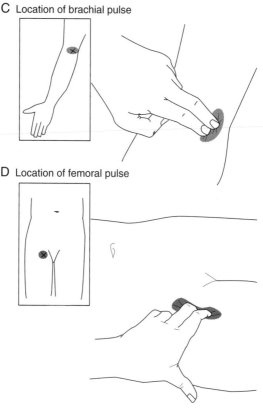

C Location of brachial pulse

D Location of femoral pulse

FIGURE 16-7 *Continued.*

E Location of popliteal pulse

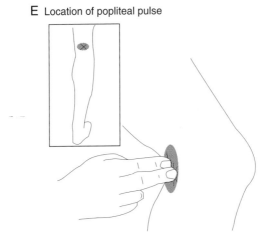

FIGURE 16-7 *Continued.*   *Illustration continued on following page*

legs 12 inches off the examining table, and ask the patient to
move the feet up and down at the ankles for approximately
1 minute. Note whether extensive pallor occurs. Next, ask
the patient to sit up and dangle the legs and feet over the
edge of the examining table. Note whether the pink color
returns to the feet, or whether they become dusky red
(rubor). Note whether there is a delay in venous return
(filling of the veins on top of the feet).

NORMAL FINDINGS	ABNORMAL FINDINGS
Blood pressure	
Will vary normally among individuals; in general, systolic pressure 95 to 140 mmHg, diastolic pressure 60 to 90 mmHg	Systolic pressure >140 mmHg or <95 mmHg; diastolic pressure >90 mmHg or <60 mmHg
Sitting Difference of 5 to 10 mmHg between both arms while sitting	Difference of >10 mmHg in both arms while sitting

F Location of dorsalis pulse

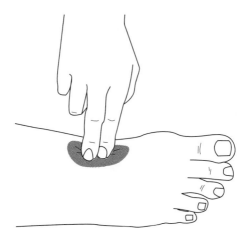

G Location of posterior tibial pulse

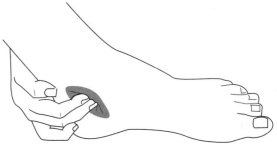

FIGURE 16-7 *Continued.*

NORMAL FINDINGS	**ABNORMAL FINDINGS**
Standing	
A systolic difference of ≤15 mmHg between both arms; diastolic difference of ≤5 mmHg between both arms	Systolic difference of >15 mmHg between both arms while standing; a diastolic difference of >5 mmHg between both arms while standing
Orthostatic changes	
Difference of <10 mmHg between sitting and standing diastolic BPs taken from the same arm	Difference of >10 mmHg between sitting and standing diastolic pressure taken from the same arm; may indicate orthostatic changes due to blood volume depletion (e.g., GI bleed)

Carotid arteries

Sixty to 90 beats/minute palpable bilaterally; strong, elastic, and regular; no bruits	A rate of <60 or >90 beats/minute, an irregular pulse, firm, inelastic, bounding pulse, alternating strength; change in the rate of the carotid pulse during inspiration (may indicate a sinus dysrhythmia); bruits, a palpable knot, or pulsating mass (requires aggressive work up to rule out thrombosis or aneurysm)

Jugular veins

Jugular venous pressure <1 inch or 2.5 cm	Jugular venous pressure <1 inch or 2.5 cm (sign of heart disease)

Peripheral venous circulation

Skin	
	Cyanosis, pallor, rubor or brownish discoloration of the lower extremities (indicates poor circulation or chronic hypoxia); slow healing lesions, ulcers, or necrotic tissue

NORMAL FINDINGS	ABNORMAL FINDINGS
Temperature Skin should be warm to touch	The temperature of the extremities is usually normal even with marked venous insufficiency
Pain No calf tenderness or pain	Tenderness along vein or in calf muscles
Sensation The patient should be able to perceive soft, sharp, and vibratory sensations	In chronic venous insufficiency, the patient may experience sensory deficits in the extremities
Vessels Veins appear bluish, feel elastic, and are nontender	Visible areas of reddening or tracking along the course of a vein; palpable tenderness, firm knots, or cords; thick, tortuous vessels; absence of sensation in an area or extremity
Edema No edema	Edema, usually ascending (beginning in the foot or ankle and progressing to the calf, knee, thigh), is a sign of venous insufficiency

Peripheral arterial circulation

Skin Normal skin (refer to Chapter 6, Assessment of the Skin, Hair, and Nails)	Presence of thin, shiny or scaly skin with decreased hair growth; thickened nails; ulcers on feet or toes that are slow to heal or progress to gangrene and necrosis
Temperature Extremities are warm to touch; temperature equal in paired extremities	Extremities are cool to touch

Pain

No pain

Tenderness or pain

Sensation

Normal sensation; able to perceive and distinguish light, dull, sharp, and vibratory sensation with eyes closed

Unable to perceive and distinguish light, dull, sharp, and vibratory sensations with eyes closed

Vessels

No bruits

Bruits while auscultating over the aorta, renal, iliac, or femoral arteries (refer to Fig. 17–4)

Edema

No edema

Edema or pitting edema

Pulse

All pulses present, strong, elastic, and regular with rating of 1+, 2+, 3+, 4+, etc.

Decreased or absent peripheral pulses

Bounding pulse: with increased pulse pressure, readily palpable, and not easily obliterated, may be secondary to exercise, anxiety, fever, atherosclerosis, hyperthyroidism

Pulsus alternans: a pulse that alternates in strength

Pulsus deferens: the pulses between the left and right extremities are different because of local circulation impairment

Clinical Notes

Be certain to palpate one carotid artery at a time so as not to potentially occlude a more distal pulse. Use light palpation because increased carotid pressure may stimulate a carotid sinus reflex and lower the heart rate and BP.

Do not overpalpate or massage suspected DVT, as this may inadvertently dislodge the thrombus and cause further harm. A duplex doppler of the lower extremities may be needed to rule out DVT, and if one is present the patient may need anticoagulant therapy.

If the patient has marked edema of the lower extremities, be certain to assess the patient's respiratory status and consider congestive heart failure.

Geriatric Considerations

	NORMAL FINDINGS
Veins	Enlargement, especially in calf veins
Pulses	Palpation of dorsalis pedis and posterior tibial pulses may be more difficult; radial artery may feel stiff, rigid, and tortuous
Orthostatic BP	Common in advanced age as a result of a decline in baroreceptor sensitivity

Clinical Notes

Falls can result from orthostatic BP changes. Carefully assess and communicate these changes to other health care professionals.

Pediatric Considerations

NORMAL FINDINGS	**ABNORMAL FINDINGS**

Newborn

Deep red, ruddy coloring
Acrocyanosis
Hands and feet cool to touch

Infant

Generalized mottling

17

Assessment of the Abdomen

HISTORY AND CURRENT STATUS QUESTIONS

Personal history of gastrointestinal, liver, gallbladder, or renal disease

Past history of liver, gallbladder, kidney, or gastrointestinal (GI) diseases such as cirrhosis, hepatitis, gallstones, renal stones, pyelonephritis, frequent urinary tract infections (UTIs), peptic ulcer disease, hiatal hernia (HH), diverticulosis, colitis, Crohn's disease, irritable bowel syndrome, or cancer (CA); history of GI bleeding (source, transfusions, surgery); alcohol consumption (amount per day)

Family history of gastrointestinal, liver, gallbladder, or renal disease

Family members with any of the problems listed above; alcohol consumption by family members

Pain?

Evaluate all complaints of pain for provocative/palliative factors, quality, region, severity, and timing (PQRST) (See Chapter 1, Table 1–1); location of the pain (referring to the four quadrants of the abdomen formed by two imaginary perpendicular lines running through the umbilicus) (see Fig. 17–1)

QUADRANT METHOD

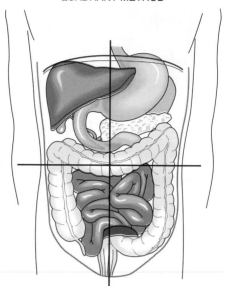

RIGHT UPPER QUADRANT (RUQ)	LEFT UPPER QUADRANT (LUQ)
Liver and gallbladder	Left liver lobe
Pylorus	Stomach
Duodenum	
Head of pancreas	Body of pancreas
Hepatic flexure of colon	Splenic flexure of colon
Portions of ascending and transverse colon	Portions of ascending and transverse colon
RIGHT LOWER QUADRANT (RLQ)	**LEFT LOWER QUADRANT (LLQ)**
Cecum and appendix	Sigmoid colon
Portion of ascending colon	Portion of descending colon

FIGURE 17–1 Abdominal quadrants.

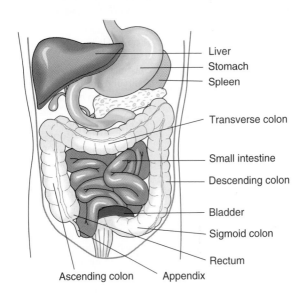

ANTERIOR VIEW OF ABDOMINAL CAVITY

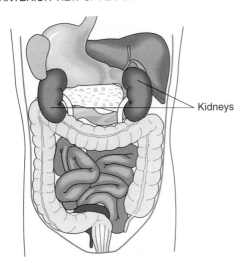

POSTERIOR VIEW OF ABDOMINAL CAVITY

FIGURE 17-2 Anatomy of the abdominal cavity.

Change in bowel habits?	Last bowel movement; change in frequency of bowel movements; constipation, straining, and difficulty moving bowels; diarrhea or urgency on moving bowels; change in the color (yellow, gray, black, blood streaked), consistency (hard, loose, watery, greasy), or shape (pencil thin or pipe stemmed) of the stool
Flatulence?	Increased belching or flatulence; diet high in gas-producing foods (onions, cabbage, carbonated beverages)
Nausea or vomiting?	Frequency, time of day, associated with eating; any food kept down without vomiting; bile, coffee grounds appearance, or hematemesis
Genitourinary symptoms?	Difficulty initiating a stream of urine, change in frequency of urination, urgency, dysuria, hematuria, pyuria, polyuria, oliguria, nocturia, leaking urine, incontinence, or stress incontinence, passage of a ureteral stone, penile or vaginal discharge?
Dysphagia?	Inability to swallow solids, liquids; frequent regurgitation after eating; bolus sensation in the throat after eating
Change in appetite?	Excessive hunger or lack of appetite (over what period of time), associated weight change
Change in weight?	Significant change in weight (how much, over what period of time)
Increasing abdominal girth?	Marked change in body habitus (increasing abdominal girth, pregnancy, ascites, tumor, impaction)

Decreased activity?   Hospitalized, wheelchair bound,
                                   depressed

Medications?   Aspirin or nonsteroidal anti-
                                   inflammatories; overuse of laxa-
                                   tives; narcotics, phenothiazides,
                                   iron, or any medications that
                                   may have increasing or decreas-
                                   ing bowel motility as a side
                                   effect

PHYSICAL EXAMINATION

Equipment

   Stethoscope
   Tape measure

Procedures, Techniques, and Findings

1. **Prepare the patient for the exam.**

   Ask the patient to undress to the waist and lie supine with
   knees slightly flexed and arms at the side or folded across
   the chest (you may need to provide pillows for the head
   and knees to make the patient more comfortable). Drape
   the upper chest to the xiphoid process and the legs and
   genitalia up to the symphysis pubis. Ask the patient to
   locate any tender areas before proceeding and examine
   these areas last. Examine the patient with warm hands
   and a warm stethoscope, distracting the patient with
   conversation while watching his facial expressions for
   confirmation of pain.

2. **Observe the patient's posture.**

   Note whether the patient is guarding or splinting the
   abdomen, lying perfectly still, constantly changing
   position, or favoring one side or position.

3. **Inspect the skin.**

   Note the color of the skin, turgor, and presence of
   erythema, ecchymosis, lesions, masses, striae, old scars, or
   venous abnormalities (refer to Chapter 6, Assessment of
   the Skin, Hair, and Nails).

4. **Inspect the abdomen.**

   Inspect the abdomen from all angles while the patient is lying supine and again while the patient holds a deep breath. Note the symmetry, the contour (flat, convex, or concave), the presence of surface movements (breathing, peristalsis, aortic pulsations), bulging or masses (hernias, cysts, tumors), obesity, and distention (obstruction, ascites) (see Fig. 17–3).

5. **Auscultate for bowel sounds.**

   Using the diaphragm of the stethoscope, auscultate the abdomen in all four quadrants formed by two imaginary lines running perpendicularly through the umbilicus (see Fig. 17–1). Begin in the left lower quadrant (LLQ) and listen for a full 5 minutes. If bowel sounds are present note their character and frequency and whether they are normal, hyperactive, or hypoactive. If they are absent, make note of this, and proceed to the other three quadrants, again auscultating in each for a full 5 minutes.

6. **Auscultate for abdominal bruits.**

   Using the bell of the stethoscope, auscultate for abdominal bruits in the target areas diagrammed (Fig. 17–4). Listen carefully for bruits, venous hums, and friction rubs in the epigastric area and all four quadrants over the aortic, renal, iliac, and femoral arteries and the thoracic aorta. If bruits are present, notify the physician of record and do not palpate the abdomen, as this may damage an existing aneurysm.

7. **Percuss the abdomen.**

   Percuss all four quadrants of the abdomen to determine the nature of underlying tissue. Hollow organs (such as the

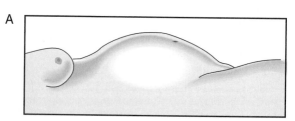

FIGURE 17-3 Abdominal profiles. A, Fully rounded or distended, umbilicus inverted.

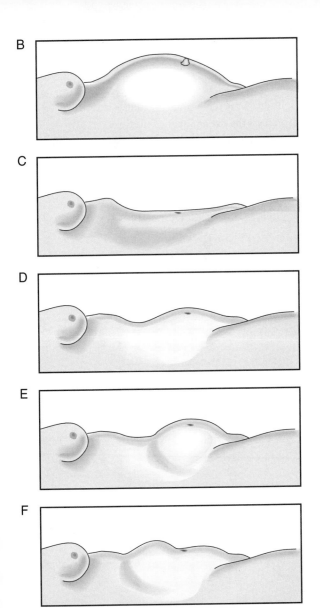

FIGURE 17-3 *Continued.* *B,* Fully rounded or distended, umbilicus everted. *C,* Scaphoid. *D,* Distended lower third. *E,* Distended lower half. *F,* Distended upper half.

gastric air bubble in the left upper quadrant, LUQ) will produce tympanic sounds, and solid or fluid-filled tissue (such as the liver, kidneys, spleen, pancreas, and distended bladder) will produce a dull sound.

8. Percuss the size and span of the liver.

Percuss upward to the lower liver edge from a point just below the umbilicus on the right midclavicular line. Mark the area where the dullness of the lower liver edge begins. Percuss downward to the upper liver edge from an area of

AUSCULTATORY LANDMARKS

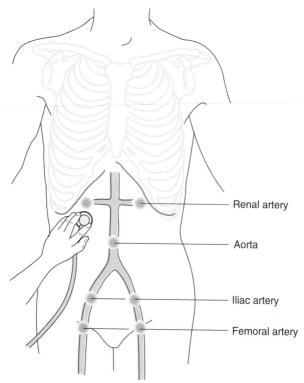

FIGURE 17-4 Auscultation for abdominal bruits.

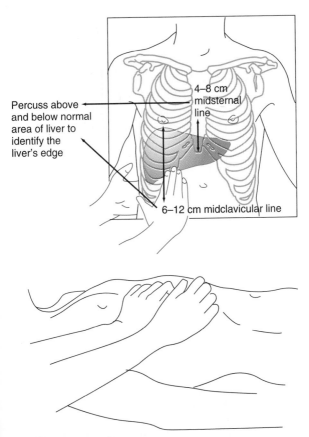

Percuss above and below normal area of liver to identify the liver's edge

4–8 cm midsternal line

6–12 cm midclavicular line

FIGURE 17-5 Measurement of the liver span.

resonant lung. Mark the area where the dullness of the upper liver edge begins. Measure between the two marks with a ruler or tape measure. This measure is the liver span (Fig. 17–5).

9. **Percuss the gastric air bubble.**

Percuss over the LUQ, the left anterior rib cage, and left epigastric area for the gastric air bubble. It will produce tympany in a small area of the LUQ (Fig. 17–6).

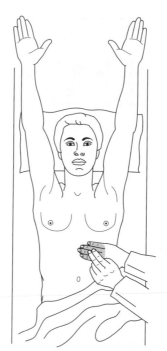

FIGURE 17-6 Percussion of the gastric air bubble.

10. Percuss the kidneys.

Ask the patient to sit or stand and percuss the posterior costovertebral angle (CVA) at the scapular line. Painless dullness should be produced over both kidneys (Fig. 17–7).

11. Percuss the spleen.

Percuss in the area of the left 10th rib just posterior to the midaxillary line. Identify the small oval area of splenic dullness. You may also percuss the normally tympanic area in lowest left interspace on the anterior axillary line. If this tympanic area grows dull when the patient takes a deep breath, the spleen may be enlarged (Fig. 17–8).

12. **Palpate the abdomen in all four quadrants using the technique of light palpation.**

    Lightly palpate the four quadrants of the abdomen to relax the patient and identify underlying organs, superficial lesions, masses, adipose tissue, and areas of increased resistance or tenderness. Palpate the abdomen with the patient supine, and again with the head slightly lifted. Use

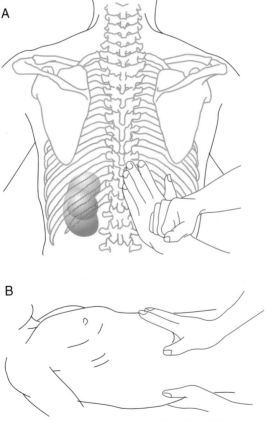

FIGURE 17-7 *A,* Percussion of kidneys. *B,* Palpation of kidneys.

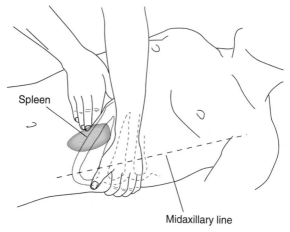

Spleen

Midaxillary line

FIGURE 17–8 Percussion of the spleen.

the fingerpads or palmar surface of three or four fingers
held together. Move methodically through each quadrant,
depressing the abdomen not more than ½ to 1 inch, while
using dipping or circular motions. Note the size, location,
and nature of any perceived abnormalities. Further
evaluate any areas of increased resistance while deliberately
distracting the patient to determine whether the resistance
is voluntary or involuntary. Palpate for rigidity of the
rectus muscles that persists despite all techniques of
relaxation.

13. **Palpate the abdomen in all four quadrants using the
technique of deep palpation. (Do not palpate deeply if
tenderness was noted on light palpation.)**

Using the palmar surface or fingerpads of three or four
fingers held together, deeply palpate the abdomen,
depressing tissue 1 to 3 inches as you move methodically
through each quadrant. Move your fingers back and forth
over underlying tissue to delineate organs and detect less
obvious masses. Never palpate over areas of tender
pulsating masses, or surgical incisions. If tenderness is
elicited, assess for the presence of rebound tenderness,
which occurs after the sudden release of deep pressure on
the abdomen.

14. Palpate the umbilicus.

Palpate the umbilicus for tenderness, masses, bulges, hernias, lesions, and discharge.

15. Palpate the liver.

Place your left hand under the patient's right posterior thorax parallel to and at the level of the 11th and 12th rib. Place your right hand on the patient's right upper quadrant (RUQ) over the midclavicular line with fingers pointing toward the head and positioned below the lower edge of liver dullness. Ask the patient to take a deep breath while pressing inward and upward with the fingers of your right hand. Attempt to feel the liver edge as it descends (see Fig. 17–5).

16. Palpate the gallbladder.

Ask the patient to take a deep breath and palpate deep below the liver margin for enlargement of the gallbladder (see Fig. 17–5) (which is normally not palpable).

17. Palpate the spleen.

Place your left hand under the patient's left CVA and your right hand on the abdomen below the left costal margin. Ask the patient to take a deep breath while you press the fingertips of your right hand inward. Palpate the edge of the spleen as it descends with inspiration (see Fig. 17–8).

18. Palpate the aorta.

Use your thumb and forefinger to palpate the aorta by pressing deeply just to the left of the verticle midline of the abdomen.

19. Palpate for ascites if the abdomen appears distended.

Ask the patient to lie supine. Have a colleague assist you by pressing his hand and forearm firmly along the vertical midline of the abdomen. Place your hands on either side of the patient's abdomen. Strike one side of the patient's abdomen forcefully with your fingertips, and with the other hand, feel for the rebounding impulse of a fluid wave (Fig. 17–9A). Another technique for determining the presence of ascites is to percuss "shifting dullness" in the abdomen. With the patient lying supine, percuss from the midline of the abdomen to the flank (Fig. 17–9B). Mark the level of dullness. Ask the patient to lie on his side and percuss again over the same area, this time from the flank

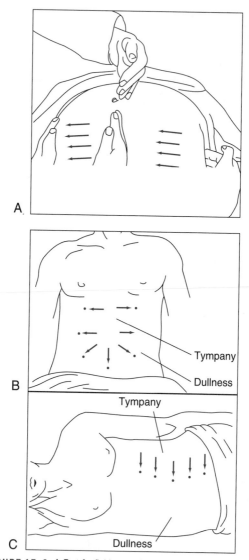

FIGURE 17-9 *A,* Test for fluid wave. *B,* Test for shifting dullness (supine). *C,* Test for shifting dullness (lying on side).

to the vertical midline of the abdomen. Note any change in the level of dullness. If ascites is present, the level of dullness will be slightly higher with the patient lying on his side (Fig. 17–9C).

20. Perform ballottement for any suspected masses.

It may be difficult to palpate a suspected mass in a patient who has significant ascites. In this situation, ballottement may prove helpful. Thrust the fingers of the right hand suddenly and forcefully into the area of the suspected mass. If the mass is freely mobile, it will initially retreat into the abdomen and immediately rebound back upward against the examiner's fingers (Fig. 17–10).

NORMAL FINDINGS	ABNORMAL FINDINGS
Posture	
Able to sit or lie comfortably and to move freely without pain in any position	Guarding, splinting, lying perfectly still, changing position frequently, leaning forward, favoring side or position
Skin	
Color consistent with the rest of the body; skin smooth, supple, without lesions, masses, or venous abnormalities (see Chapter 6, Assessment of the Skin, Hair, and Nails)	Presence of erythema, ecchymosis, lesions, masses, edema, old surgical scars, venous abnormalities, or markedly diminished or excessive adipose tissue; jaundice, or a yellow hue to the skin and sclera, may indicate underlying liver or gallbladder disease; a glistening taut abdomen may indicate the presence of ascites; a bluish tinge to the abdomen (Cullen's sign) may indicate internal bleeding; bruising of the flank, or Grey Turner's sign, may indicate pancreatitis or internal bleeding

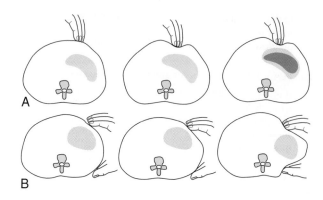

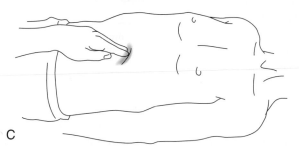

LIGHT BALLOTTEMENT

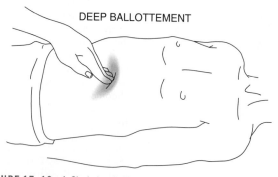

DEEP BALLOTTEMENT

FIGURE 17-10 *A,* Single-handed ballottement. *B,* Bimanual ballottement. *C,* Light ballottement. *D,* Deep ballottement.

NORMAL FINDINGS	ABNORMAL FINDINGS

Abdomen

Soft, smooth, consistent, symmetrical, and nontender; flat, convex, or (in thin people) concave; mild distention normally below the umbilicus secondary to a full bladder or stool in the colon; tympany should be percussed over the gastric air bubble and gas-filled bowel; dullness should be percussed over all other underlying organs; light palpation should elicit no tenderness, guarding, or masses; deep palpation may elicit tenderness normally over the xiphoid process, cecum, and sigmoid colon; the abdomen may be symmetrically distended after eating a heavy meal, or in obese patients

Involuntary guarding, a tender, rigid, or boardlike abdomen, or the presence of rebound tenderness usually indicates an acute process; asymmetry above the umbilicus; asymmetry below the umbilicus; abnormal distention of the abdomen occurs with the accumulation of fluid, feces, gas, or tumor

Bowel sounds

High pitched, irregular gurgling sounds as gas passes through the bowel; singularly or in clusters, last ½ to several seconds, occur at a rate of 1 to 35/minute; normally do not occur in all four quadrants, but should occur in at least one; hyperactive bowel sounds in patients who are hungry or who have just eaten

Hyperactive bowel sounds (borborygmy) in response to inflammation of the bowel, laxative abuse or overuse, and certain spicy foods; hypoactive bowel sounds or the complete cessation of bowel sounds in response to conditions that decrease the gastric motility

Text continued on page 303

TABLE 17-1 Common Variations and Abnormalities of the Abdomen

Variation	Description Significance	Quality of Pain Localization	Aggravating and Relieving Factors	Physical Signs	Diagnostic Tests
Hernia					
Bowel obstruction	Obstruction of the bowel either by stricture, mass, necrotic tissue, intussusception, or fecal impaction	Abdominal pain will depend on location of obstruction Usually pain will be in lower abdomen with large bowel obstruction and periumbilical with small bowel obstruction	May be aggravated by food May be relieved by vomiting, or decompression with nasogastric tube to gravity or low suction	Distended abdomen Decreased bowel sounds May be accompanied by projectile vomiting and fecal odor to emesis	Abdominal flat plate and upright will show air fluid levels in bowel
Hiatal hernia	A portion of the stomach herniates up through the diaphragm	Burning epigastric and hypogastric pain	Pain may be exacerbated by lying flat and relieved by sitting more upright at a 45° angle Elevating the head of the bed often helps to relieve pain at night		Barium swallow, upper endoscopy, abdominal ultrasound

Gastric ulcer	A lesion in the lining of the stomach	Usually burning periumbilical or hypogastric pain. In the case of perforation, severe pain of sudden onset which may radiate to the shoulder	Exacerbated by eating. In case of perforation, pain may worsen with movement	If bleeding, melena Stool positive for occult blood	Barium swallow, upper endoscopy
Duodenal ulcer	Lesion in the duodenum	Burning periumbilical or hypogastric abdominal pain	Exacerbated by eating; pain may occur ½–1 hour after eating	If bleeding may find melena, or stool positive for occult blood	Barium swallow, upper endoscopy
Cholelithiasis	Calculi or stones in the gallbladder	Crampy, sometimes moderate to severe pain in the RUQ (right upper quadrant)	Exacerbated by fatty food consumption Relieved by cholecystectomy	Tenderness and sometimes a fullness of the RUQ (right upper quadrant)	Ultrasound, ERCP
Cholecystitis	Inflammation or infection of the gallbladder	Moderate to severe RUQ (right upper quadrant) pain which may radiate to the right shoulder and scapula	Relieved by antibiotics or cholecystectomy	Fever, chills, rigors	Ultrasound, HIDA scan

Table continued on following page

TABLE 17-1	Common Variations and Abnormalities of the Abdomen *Continued*				
Variation	Description Significance	Quality of Pain Localization	Aggravating and Relieving Factors	Physical Signs	Diagnostic Tests
Pancreatitis	Inflammation or infection of the pancreas	Severe constant epigastric tenderness, may have rebound tenderness Pain may radiate to the back	Exacerbated by alcohol consumption May occur post ERCP Pain often relieved by sitting forward Relieved with antibiotics	Epigastric tenderness, fever	Elevated serum amylase
Hepatitis	Inflammation or infection of the liver	Tenderness in the RUQ (right upper quadrant)		RUQ tenderness with malaise Nausea, vomiting, fever, jaundice	Serum hepatitis screening Liver biopsy
Cirrhosis			Alcohol consumption can cause an aggravated cirrhosis	Enlarged liver with firm nontender edge	Liver biopsy

Abdominal aortic aneurysm	A weakening of the abdominal aortic wall with subsequent ballooning out of a thinner-walled pocket at risk for rupture	Pulsatile mass in midabdomen may become tender when threatening to rupture, and once ruptured may become rigid and have a mottled appearance	Exacerbated by anticoagulant therapy	Pulsatile mass in midabdomen. May be accompanied by severe pain radiating to the back, rigid abdomen, hypotension, and shock if ruptured	Ultrasound of the abdomen. Angiography. A calcified aneurysm may be revealed by abdominal x-ray
Appendicitis	Inflammation or infection of the appendix	Initially periumbilical pain that later localizes to the right lower quadrant with classic rebound tenderness	Exacerbated by movement. Usually the rectal exam is painful	Fever, tenderness, and guarding in the right iliac fossa (right lower quadrant)	Ultrasound, surgery, laparoscopy
Renal/ureteral calculi	Formation of calculi (stones) in the renal pelvis which may send small pieces down the ureters	Severe colicky pain in flank and loins which causes the patient to writhe and attempt to frequently change position	Exacerbated by dehydration	May be accompanied by fever, nausea, vomiting, obstruction, or urinary retention. May have pain on first palpation of costovertebral angle (costovertebral angle tenderness)	Ultrasound of kidneys, urethra, and bladder. Abdominal x-ray may show calculi. Intravenous urogram

Table continued on following page

	TABLE 17-1 Common Variations and Abnormalities of the Abdomen *Continued*				
Variation	Description Significance	Quality of Pain Localization	Aggravating and Relieving Factors	Physical Signs	Diagnostic Tests
Pyelonephritis	Inflammation or infection of the kidneys	Costovertebral angle tenderness	Exacerbated by dehydration Relieved by hydration and antibiotics	May be accompanied by fever, malaise, nausea, vomiting	Urinalysis and urine culture
Diverticulosis	Outpocketing of sections of the colon	Crampy pain in LLQ (left lower quadrant)	Relieved by consumption of food high in fiber		Colonoscopy Barium enema
Diverticulitis	Inflammation or infection of a diverticula	Crampy to severe LLQ pain	Relieved by antibiotics	Fever, malaise, diarrhea	Colonoscopy Barium enema
Colon cancer	Malignancy, mass, in lining of the colon	Oftentimes painless	Relieved by surgery	Malaise, anorexia, anemia, weight loss in later stages Occult blood in stool	Colonoscopy and biopsy

Condition	Description	Pain	Treatment	Symptoms	Diagnostic Tests
Ectopic pregnancy	Extrauterine pregnancy, either in the ovarian tubes, ovaries, or abdominal cavity	Becomes painful as it nears rupture between 6–8 weeks gestational age Pain is severe, usually unilateral low abdominal pain	Relieved by surgery Exacerbated by movement	Positive pregnancy test May be accompanied by nausea, vomiting, vaginal spotting or bleeding	Positive pregnancy test Ultrasound of the abdomen
Endometritis	Inflammation or infection of the endometrium	Bilateral low abdominal pain	Antibiotics		Hysteroscopy with biopsy
Pelvic inflammatory disease	Infection of the pelvis, uterus, or fallopian tubes	Severe bilateral low abdominal pain	Exacerbated by unprotected vaginal intercourse Pain exacerbated by walking and moving Relieved by antibiotics	Severe bilateral low abdominal pain with vaginal discharge and cervical motion tenderness	Vaginal and cervical cultures

Table continued on following page

301

TABLE 17-1 Common Variations and Abnormalities of the Abdomen *Continued*

Variation	Description Significance	Quality of Pain Localization	Aggravating and Relieving Factors	Physical Signs	Diagnostic Tests
Pelvic/adnexal mass	Malignancy of the uterus, fallopian tube, or ovary	May be painless	Exacerbated by immunosuppression, pregnancy	There may be no accompanying symptoms There may be weight loss, anorexia, nausea, vomiting, anemia, fullness, or heaviness in low abdomen There may be urinary retention or obstruction	Ultrasound or CT scan of pelvis
Tubo-ovarian abscess/cyst	Fluid or blood filled abscess on the fallopian tube or ovary	Crampy, colicky unilateral low abdominal pain May become severe if abscess or cyst ruptures	Exacerbated by movement Relieved by surgery	Crampy or colicky unilateral pain May be accompanied by fever, chills, nausea, or vomiting	Ultrasound Laparoscopy

NORMAL FINDINGS	ABNORMAL FINDINGS
Bruits	
No bruits should be heard	Bruits, venous hums, or friction rubs; *do not palpate the abdomen if bruits are heard,* as this may damage an existing aneurysm
Umbilicus	
Free of lesions, masses, hernias, and discharge	An umbilical hernia may cause protrusion or displacement of the umbilicus; tenderness, erythema or discharge may indicate infection or abscess
Stomach	
A tympanic area corresponding to the gastric air bubble usually percussed in the left upper quadrant	
Liver	
Dull to percussion; span normally 6 to 12 cm (2½ to 5 inches); lower edge often not palpable, however, when palpable, should be smooth, firm, regular, and nontender; liver edge may normally descend up to 1 inch on deep inspiration	Enlarged liver span (>12 cm), irregular contour, or tenderness on deep palpation
Gallbladder	
Nontender and usually not palpable	Enlarged, palpable, tender gallbladder; a positive Murphy's sign, or abrupt cessation of inspiration while deeply palpating the gallbladder, indicative of an acute process

NORMAL FINDINGS	ABNORMAL FINDINGS
Kidneys	
Dull to percussion, not palpable, no CVA tenderness	CVA tenderness; enlarged, palpable kidneys
Spleen	
Dull to percussion, and nontender; not palpable	Change from tympany to dullness while percussing the lowest left interspace as the patient takes a deep breath; enlarged, palpable, or tender spleen
Aorta	
Usually palpable (unless the patient is morbidly obese) with strong and regular pulsations	Faint or irregular pulsations; pulsating mass may indicate an aneurysm (which should never be further palpated to avoid inflicting damage)

Clinical Notes

Current studies refute past beliefs that analgesics should not be administered to patients with acute abdominal pain prior to physical assessment on the premise that analgesia will mask physical findings. In fact the contrary has been shown to be true, that analgesia has actually helped patients to relax, and has allowed more accurate localization of pain.

Never palpate an abdomen if bruits are present or a pulsating mass has been detected on light palpation. Deep palpation may cause damage to an underlying aneurysm.

Patients presenting with abdominal pain, or alteration in bowel habits, should be given a digital rectal exam, (refer to Chapter 20, Assessment of the Anus, Rectum, and Prostate) and have their stool tested for occult blood.

Special care should be taken when examining pregnant women to differentiate what may be common symptoms associated with pregnancy from possible underlying GI disease.

Some acute conditions of the abdomen (ectopic pregnancy, ruptured cyst) may produce referred pain to the shoulder.

Patients may present initially with complaints of severe shoulder pain similar in nature to bursitis.

Geriatric Considerations

	NORMAL FINDINGS
Abdominal wall	Weakened abdominal muscle tone
	Accumulation of fat in lower abdomen
Bowel sounds	Slowed intestinal motility
Liver	Palpation will be easier

Clinical Notes

Changes attributable to aging often enhance palpation of abdominal organs. A mass of stool in the descending or sigmoid colon can be mistaken for malignancy. Treatment of constipation and reexamination are indicated.

The supine position may be uncomfortable for the older patient. Place a pillow under the head and knees to promote comfort.

Pediatric Considerations

Physical Examination

PROCEDURE

May place child's hand beneath examiner's to reduce ticklishness.

NORMAL FINDINGS	ABNORMAL FINDINGS
Newborn	
Umbilical cord may fall off in 1 to 2 weeks	
Umbilical granuloma	Hard stools
Umbilical hernia	
Diastasis recti	
Infant	
Protuberant abdomen	
	Concave abdomen
Liver edge smooth and palpable 1 to 3 cm below RUQ	
Epigastric pulsations	Pyloric stenosis: projectile vomiting, olive-sized mass in RUQ

NORMAL FINDINGS	ABNORMAL FINDINGS
Spleen tip palpable	
Bladder palpable above symphysis pubis	
	Intussusception: intermittent pain with current jelly stool
Abdominal breathing pattern	

Child

	Hirschprung's disease: megacolon, pencil-thin stools
Protuberant abdomen when erect, flat when supine	
Superficial venous pattern	Dilated veins

Clinical Notes

Flexing hips and knees relaxes the abdomen.

Abdominal pain is usually diffuse and general in children, making it difficult to localize inflammation.

Ask child to lift chair in which examiner sits to visualize a hernia.

RAPID ASSESSMENT

THE PATIENT WITH ABDOMINAL PAIN

What is the quality of the pain—burning, sharp, dull, aching, crushing?

Pressure, as though someone were standing on your chest, or universal sign of the clenched fist?

Is the pain diffuse or localized? (RUQ, hypogastric, periumbilical, flank, RLQ, LLQ, suprapubic, sacral pain)

Does the pain move about or change location? Does the pain radiate? Occur before or after eating?

Is the abdomen distended?

Are there normal, hypoactive, hyperactive or absent bowel sounds?

Are there audible bruits?

Is the pain elicited on palpation—light or deep?

Is there rebound tenderness?

Are there any associated symptoms of nausea, vomiting, diarrhea, fever, constipation flatulence, jaundice?

Has the patient experienced a change in bowel habits—constipation, diarrhea, tenesmus, melena, bright red blood per rectum, steatorrhea, gray yellow or black stools?

Is there dysuria, pyuria, penile or vaginal discharge?

Is there an enlarged or tender prostate?

Is there cervical motion tenderness or discharge on pelvic exam?

Is there an enlarged uterus or palpable adnexal tenderness fullness or masses?

Physical Examination	Rationale
Check vital signs.	Determine presence of fever (infectious process, flue, gastroenteritis, peritonitis, pylonephritis, cholecystitis, urinary tract infection). Determine orthostatic blood pressure (acute blood loss, GI bleed, perforated gallbladder, appendicitis, diverticula, esophageal varices rupture, aneurysm) Determine pulse tachycardia, bradycardia. Determine respiratory rate—tachypnea
Observe abdomen for abnormal contours.	Determine presence of distention, due to hernia, obstruction, ascites, urinary retention, aneurysm.
Auscultate the abdomen for abnormal bowel sounds and bruits.	Bruits may be present in renal artery occlusion, aortic aneurysm, femoral artery occlusion.

Continued on next page

Physical Examination	Rationale
Palpate the abdomen for tenderness and masses	Determine whether there is localized tenderness. RUQ: Hepatitis, cholecystitis, gallstones, liver abcess. Periumbilical; gastroenteritis, appendicitis. RLQ: appendicitis, Tubo-ovarian abscess, ectopic pregnancy. LLQ: tubo-ovarian abscess, ectopic pregnancy, diverticulitiis. Suprabupic: Urinary tract infection, cystitis
Palpate the liver edge	Determine whether the liver is tender (hepatitis, abscess, infection, laceration)
Percuss the liver size	Determine whether the liver is enlarged due to an abcess or mass
Palpate the spleen	Determine whether the spleen is tender or enlarged
Palpate the kidneys	Determine whether there are palpable masses or tenderness (polycystic kidneys, renal cyst, mass)
Percuss the bladder	Suprabupic tenderness may indicate urinary tract infection or cystitis
Perform a pelvic exam	Determine whether there is vaginal or cervical discharge, cervical motion tenderness (PID) or presence of uterine or adnexal masses
Perform a rectal exam including examination of the prostate in males	Determine whether prostate is enlarged or tender. An enlarged prostate may cause urinary retention or obstruction. A tender prostate may indicate infection.
Examine the stool and perform a stool guaiac test	The presence of blood in the stool may indicate a GI bleed.

Assessment of the Female Genitalia 18

HISTORY AND CURRENT STATUS QUESTIONS

Personal sexual history

Note sexual orientation (heterosexual, homosexual, bisexual); type of sexual activity engaged in (vaginal, oral, or anal intercourse); frequency of sexual activity; number of partners; "safer sex" practices and condom use; risky practices; previous sexually transmitted diseases (STDs) (when, how treated, tested for cure); recent exposure to a partner with an STD, hepatitis B, or human immunodeficiencey virus (HIV); other risk factors for hepatitis B or HIV; partner tested or treated for either of these

Obstetric history

Note the patient's obstetric history (written G—P_ _ _ _); list in order total number of pregnancies (G), and total number of births, (P) number of premature births, number of abortions (spontaneous and elective combined), and number of living children

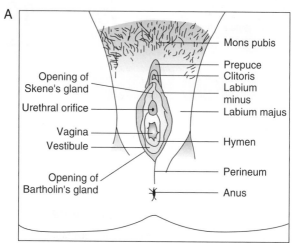

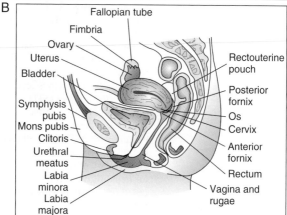

FIGURE 18-1 Anatomy of the female genitalia. *A*, Exterior view. *B*, Interior view.

| Menstrual history | Record the patient's menstrual "triad": age of onset of menses, usual number of days duration, and usual length of the menstrual cycle in days; note the |

	LMP, or date of the last menstrual period; note whether the patient reports any premenstrual symptoms of headache, dizziness, cramping, fatigue, anxiety
Menstrual irregularity?	LMP (regular, on time) prior periods regular; missed period (amenorrhea); painful periods (dysmenorrhea), unusually heavy bleeding (menorrhagia), or intermenstrual bleeding or spotting (metrorrhagia); other symptoms associated with menses (headache, fatigue, dizziness, nausea, vomiting, anxiety, premenstrual syndrome)
Pregnancy?	Pain, spotting, discharge, cessation of fetal movement, breast tenderness, nausea, lightheadedness, weight change; recent pregnancy test and type (urine or blood, positive or negative); last vaginal intercourse; birth control method used
Birth control?	Method (be as specific as possible, including brand names); past failure problems associated with the use of current or previous methods; recent change of method; known contraindications to any particular method
Pruritis?	Localized or diffuse, location; associated lesions, erythema, excoriations
Infestations?	Lice, scabies, fleas; recent exposure; parasites or nits seen
Lesions?	Type (macule, papule, ulcer, vesicle, rash, laceration, excoriation), number (single or in clusters), location (vulva, labia, vaginal wall, cervix, anus), distri-

	bution (symmetrical or asymmetrical), pain, pruritis, suppuration
Discharge?	Characteristics (scant, profuse, thick, thin, frothy, malodorous, clear, white, gray, yellow, green); constant or intermittent; relation to the menstrual cycle (during ovulation; prior to, during, or after menses)
Pain?	Type (low abdominal or back pain, diffuse or localized); provocative/palliative factors, quality, region, severity, timing (PQRST)
Genitourinary symptoms?	Increased urinary frequency, urgency, dysuria, hematuria, pyuria, polyuria, oliguria, nocturia, incontinence, or stress incontinence; duration of symptoms; associated symptoms (fever, flank pain, abdominal pain, nausea, or vomiting)
Masses or swelling?	Labial edema, Bartholin's cyst or abscess, cystocele, rectocele, uterine prolapse; vulvar, vaginal, cervical cancer; painful or nontender; purulent or draining
Infertility?	Previous pregnancy; time spent "trying" to get pregnant without success; fertility workup (patient and partner), results
Sexual dysfunction?	Loss of libido, loss of orgasm, vaginal atrophy, loss of lubrication, vaginismus, or painful coitus; feelings of ambivalence, insecurity, anxiety, or depression with regard to current relationships
Sexual assault?	Evaluation and counselling by an experienced crisis team

PHYSICAL EXAMINATION
Equipment

Gyn examining table

Gooseneck lamp

Gown

Drape

Gloves

Speculum

Culturettes (both viral and bacterial)

Microscope slides

Normal saline

Potassium hydroxide (KOH)

Papanicoulou (PAP) test scrapers

Procedures, Techniques, and Findings

1. **Prepare patient and materials for examination.**

   Ask the patient to urinate and empty her bladder. Have her undress from the waist down and assume a semirecumbent position on the examining table with her knees and thighs draped and her feet in the stirrups. Ask the patient to rest her hands on her waist, relax her knees, and let them fall to the side as far as possible.

2. **Inspect and palpate the vulva for lesions, masses, and abnormalities.**

   Touch the patient's thigh initially to avoid startling her, then proceed with the exam, parting the pubic hair as necessary to facilitate thorough examination. Palpate any noticeable masses, lesions, swelling or abnormalities.

3. **Inspect the pubic hair for infestations, density of growth, and sexual maturity.**

   Part the pubic hair to look for infestations of pubic lice often found at the base of the pubic hair. Search also for nits adhered to the hair stalks. Assess the sexual maturity of the patient (Fig. 18–2).

4. **Inspect and palpate the labia majora for lesions, masses, inflammation, swelling, and abnormalities.**

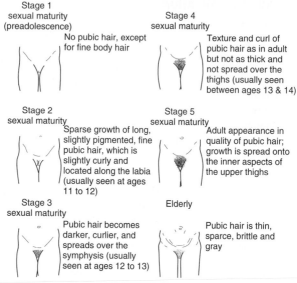

Stage 1
sexual maturity
(preadolescence)
No pubic hair, except
for fine body hair

Stage 4
sexual maturity
Texture and curl of
pubic hair as in adult
but not as thick and
not spread over the
thighs (usually seen
between ages 13 & 14)

Stage 2
sexual maturity
Sparse growth of long,
slightly pigmented, fine
pubic hair, which is
slightly curly and
located along the labia
(usually seen at ages
11 to 12)

Stage 5
sexual maturity
Adult appearance in
quality of pubic hair;
growth is spread onto
the inner aspects of
the upper thighs

Stage 3
sexual maturity
Pubic hair becomes
darker, curlier, and
spreads over the
symphysis (usually
seen at ages 12 to 13)

Elderly
Pubic hair is thin,
sparce, brittle and
gray

FIGURE 18-2 Stages of female sexual maturity.

Inspect and palpate with one or two fingers any lesions, masses, or abnormalities. You may need to grasp the labia between two fingers to accomplish a thorough examination.

5. **Inspect the labia minora for position, lesions, masses, or abnormalities.**

   Separate the labia majora with your gloved fingers, and inspect the labia minora for lesions, masses, inflammation, swelling, and abnormalities. Palpate all noticed lesions thoroughly.

6. **Inspect the clitoris for position, size, lesions, masses, and abnormalities.**

   Locate the clitoris between the anterior junction of the labia majora and the labia minora. Inspect and palpate for lesions, masses, enlargement, and abnormalities.

7. **Inspect the urethral meatus and Skene's glands for lesions, masses, inflammation, discharge, or abnormalities.**

Separate the labia minora and locate the urethral meatus, a small orifice just below the anterior junction of the labia minora. Inspect for lesions, masses, discharge, and abnormalities (Fig. 18–3A). If there is inflammation or urethritis is suspected, milk the urethra gently by inserting a gloved finger into the vagina and stroking its posterior side in a downward motion toward you. Culture any discharge for bacteria, gonorrhea, and chlamydia.

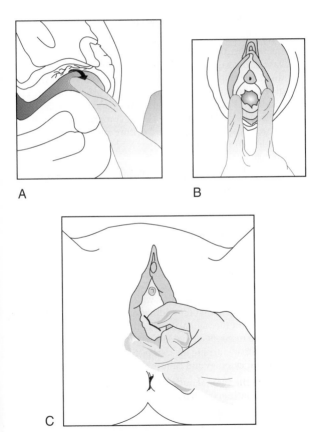

A   B

C

FIGURE 18-3 Vaginal examination. *A,* Palpation of Skene's glands. *B,* Inspection of hymen and vaginal introitus. *C,* Palpation of Bartholin's glands.

8. **Inspect the hymen and note whether it is intact. Inspect the vaginal introitus or vaginal opening for lesions, masses, inflammation, tears, discharge, and support.**

   Inspect the hymen and vaginal introitus. The hymen may be intact in children and virgins. Inspect for lesions, masses, inflammation, and tears (Fig. 18–3B). Palpate any abnormalities. With the labia separated by your gloved finger, ask the patient to bear down to allow the support of the vaginal outlet to be evaluated. Observe and note any abnormal bulging or swelling.

9. **Inspect the Bartholin's glands for pain, swelling, masses, or discharge.**

   Inspect the Bartholin's glands, located bilaterally at the base of the vaginal opening, for pain, swelling, masses, and discharge (Fig. 18–3C). Palpate the glands between your gloved index finger and your thumb by placing one finger inside the base of the vaginal opening and one on the outside of the labia majora. Gently compress the glands between your two fingers and culture any discharge exuding from the duct openings for bacteria, gonorrhea, and chlamydia.

10. **Inspect the cervix and cervical os for position, shape, size, color, inflammation, erythema, lesions, masses, and discharge.**

    Lubricate your gloved fingers and speculum with water. Insert one or two fingers into the vaginal opening and press downward on the posterior aspect in order to further open the introitus and facilitate the insertion of the speculum. With the speculum closed and held so that the blade width is in a verticle position, insert the speculum. Gently push in a downward sloping fashion, while at the same time rotating the blade so that the width is now in a horizontal position. Follow the vaginal canal to the cervix. Open the speculum and manipulate the cervix into position and secure the speculum by turning the clamp (Fig. 18–4). Obtain specimens for cytology and culture any discharge (Fig. 18–5).

11. **Inspect the vaginal outlet for lesions, masses, inflammation, discharge, and abnormalities.**

    Unclamp the speculum and hold it open as you withdraw it slowly from the vaginal canal. As you withdraw the speculum inspect the walls of the vaginal canal. Use a

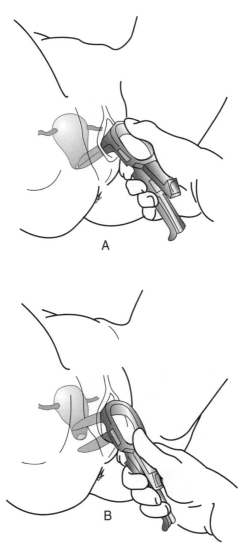

FIGURE 18-4 Vaginal examination. *A*, Insertion of the speculum. *B*, Opening of the speculum blades.

gooseneck lamp or pen light to better illuminate the
canal.

12. Palpate the vaginal wall for masses, lesions, and abnormalities.

Lubricate the index and middle finger of a gloved right
hand. Insert the two fingers into the vagina. Palpate the
anterior, posterior, and lateral walls of the vaginal
canal.

13. Palpate the cervix for position, shape, size, consistency. Determine whether the cervical os is open or closed.

Palpate the cervix with the tips of your fingers. Note
position, shape, consistency, and mobility of the cervix.
Gently move the cervix from side to side and test for
cervical motion tenderness (Fig. 18–6A). Attempt to admit
one fingertip into the cervical os. Usually the os is closed
and you will feel tight resistance. If it admits one fingertip,
or offers no resistance, it is considered open.

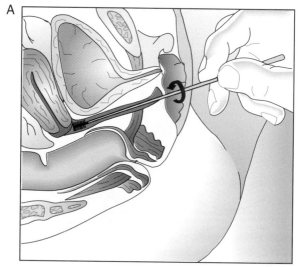

FIGURE 18-5 *A,* Obtaining a cervical smear.

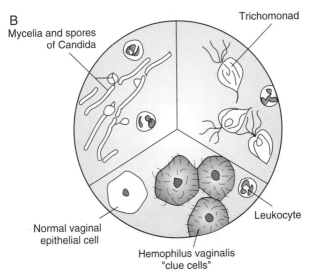

FIGURE 18–5 Continued. B, Microscopic appearance of vaginal microorganisms.

14. **Palpate the ovaries and adnexa.**

    Place your left hand on the patient's abdomen about halfway between the umbilicus and the symphysis pubis. Push inward and downward toward the symphysis pubis while at the same time pushing upward on the vaginal mucosa lateral to the cervix with the fingers of your right hand. Try to palpate the small almond-shaped ovary on either side (Fig. 18–6B). Palpate for the adnexa. Normally it will not be palpable unless there is adnexal thickening.

15. **Palpate the uterus for position, size, shape, consistency.**

    With your hands positioned as described above, push downward toward the symphysis pubis with your left hand while pushing upward on the cervix with the fingers of your right hand. Attempt to grasp the uterus between the fingers of your two hands (Fig. 18–6). Note the position, size, shape, consistency, and mobility of the uterus. Note also whether the uterus is tender.

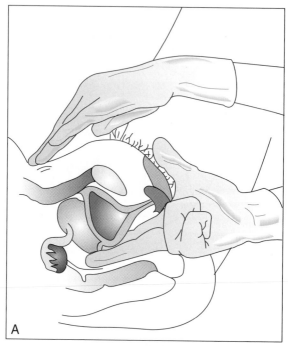

FIGURE 18-6 *A,* Bimanual palpation of the uterus.

NORMAL FINDINGS	ABNORMAL FINDINGS
Vulva	
Skin	
Smooth, warm skin; pink in light-skinned people and olive to brown in dark-skinned people. May be lighter in color than the rest of the body because of lack of exposure to sun	Red, hot, erythematous; ecchymosis, hematomas, irregular pigment
Lesions	
None	Excoriations, masses, papules, macules, vesicles, ulcers, rash, or wheals

Infestations

None	Lice, scabies, fleas

Pubic hair

Quantity and distribution of pubic hair should be consistent with the sexual maturity expected for the patient's age

Abnormal distribution for age may indicate hormonal imbalances, chronic disease, dermatitis, or response to medication; hair loss may be symmetrical and nonscarring or asymmetrical and scarring

Infestations

None

Lice usually found at the base of the pubic hairs; nits found adhered to the hair stalks

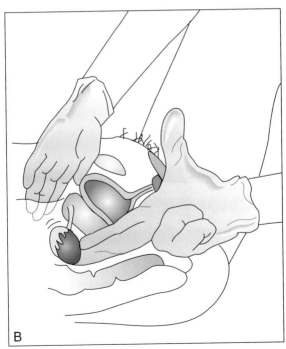

FIGURE 18-6 *Continued.* *B,* Bimanual palpation of the adnexa.

NORMAL FINDINGS	ABNORMAL FINDINGS

Labia majora

Smooth, moist skin, without lesions, ecchymosis, erythema; usually symmetrical in size and shape; lie together in children and virgins and remain parted open in sexually active women and after childbirth; skin on the inner aspect may be slightly darker	Red, hot, dry, skin; edema, erythema, ecchymosis, tears, lacerations; lesions such as macules, papules, vesicles, ulcers, venereal warts, masses; tenderness

Clitoris

Normally pink without lesions; size does not exceed 2 cm in length by 0.5 cm in width	Bright red color, erythema, ecchymosis, lesions; enlarged clitoris may indicate hormonal or developmental masculinization *May also be excised in some religious and cultural groups*

Urethral meatus

Located midline and anterior to the vaginal opening; pink with a slitlike opening; without lesions, discharge, tenderness	Red, erythematous; prolapse, polyps, fistula, lesions, discharge, edema, tenderness

Hymen

May be intact in virgins and restrict the opening of the vagina; in sexually active women only remnants of the hymen remain	If edematous, torn, or absent in small children sexual abuse must be considered

Introitus

Usually open and unobstructed	Obstructed by a cystocele, a bulging mass descending from the anterior vaginal wall, or by a rectocele, arising from the posterior

vaginal floor; usually caused by inadequate support of the vaginal outlet; a large smooth pink protruding tissue mass may actually be a uterine prolapse with the cervix visible in the vaginal canal

Bartholin's glands

Normally nontender, and not palpable	Large nontender unilateral mass may be a Bartholin's cyst; a large, hot, tender, fluctuant mass, either unilateral or bilateral may be a Bartholin's abscess; abscess may be fluctuant, have tracked, or have spontaneously ruptured
	Discharge from the site may culture positive for gonorrhea, or chlamydia

Vaginal wall

Ruggated homogenous tissue, with thin clear or cloudy odorless secretions; secretions usually increased in pregnancy; no lesions or masses	Thick, curdlike, or foul-smelling discharge; lesions, masses, vesicles, papules, warts

Cervix

Usually pink, smooth, moist, glistening, rounded, firm mass, approximately 1 inch in diameter; may be enlarged, soft, and blue tinged in pregnancy, and pale during menopause; os is usually a central depression with a rounded opening in nulliparous women, and a "fish-mouthed" opening in multiparous women; no dis-	Erythema, lesions, discharge, friable surface, bleeding (between periods), lacerations, polyps, prolapse or enlargement of the cervix are abnormal findings; an open cervical os may indicate threatened abortion or incompetent cervix; lesions may indicate STD (papules, venereal warts; vesicles, herpes simplex II; ulcers,

NORMAL FINDINGS	ABNORMAL FINDINGS
charge, lesions, masses, erythema, or cervical motion tenderness are present	either primary syphilis or chancroid; macules, secondary syphilis)

Uterus

Usually firm, nontender, "6-week"-size mass in the nonpregnant female; contour should be smooth, regular, without palpable nodules or masses	Enlarged, soft, or tender; may indicate pregnancy, fibroids, hydatidiform mole, or mass

Clinical Notes

Male practitioners should always be accompanied by a chaperone throughout the course of the examination. Female practitioners should be accompanied by a chaperone if the patient is emotionally unstable.

A thorough gyn exam should include a Pap smear for cytology, cultures for gonorrhea and chlamydia, and a wet prep and KOH for trichomonas and yeast.

A VDRL should be sent on all patients as part of their annual gyn check, and whenever diagnosing or screening for STDs.

A pregnancy test should be sent on all women of childbearing age who complain of vaginal bleeding, low abdominal pain, discharge, or any abnormality of their menstrual cycle.

Choose an appropriate type and size of speculum for the age of patient being examined. Test the clamping device and thumb screws to be sure they are working properly before inserting the speculum into the patient's vagina.

Geriatric Considerations

	NORMAL FINDINGS
Pubic hair	Thin, sparse, and gray
Uterus	Diminished in size
Ovaries	Diminished in size, often not palpable
Labia	Thin, flattened appearance
Vagina	Shorten and narrow in structure; mucosa dry, thin, and pale.

Clinical Notes

A weakening of the pelvic floor musculature may result in protrusion of the bladder (cystocele) or protrusion of the rectum (rectocele) into the vagina.

Dwindling hormones and age-related changes in the pelvic floor and bladder contribute to urge incontinence in the older female patient. Obtain a clear, complete history of voiding patterns.

Pelvic examination in a postmenopausal sexually inactive woman may need to be modified to a single-digit examination.

 Pediatric Considerations

History

Bubble baths?

Cotton or other underwear?

Masturbation behaviors?

Known sexual abuse?

Development of secondary sexual characteristics?

Age of menarche? Regular cycle? Dysmenorrhea?

Sexually active? Known to family or confidential?

Knowledge base re: contraception and STDs?

Conflicts re: sexual identity/orientation?

Physical Examination

PROCEDURE. To examine the external genitalia, gently retract the labia; having a small child cough may expose the vaginal mucosa for better visualization.

NORMAL FINDINGS	ABNORMAL FINDINGS
Infant	
Labia minora prominent Edema, bruising of genitals post delivery Bloody or serosanguinous vaginal discharge	Ambiguous genitalia

NORMAL FINDINGS	ABNORMAL FINDINGS

Infant and child

Labia minora atrophy; almost nonexistent until puberty

Perianal skin tags	Vaginal discharge
Partially fused labia	Near complete fusion of labia obstructing urinary flow
Secondary sexual characteristics as early as the 8th year	

Clinical Notes

Refer to Tanner staging (see Chapter 13) to determine degree of sexual maturation.

Menstrual cycle may be irregular for 2 years postmenarche.

Secondary amenorrhea for 6 months or less, in the absence of other signs of disease, is of no serious concern in the adolescent.

Assessment of the Male Genitalia 19

HISTORY AND CURRENT STATUS QUESTIONS

Personal sexual history	Sexual orientation (heterosexual, homosexual, bisexual), type of sexual activity engaged in (vaginal, oral, anal intercourse), frequency of sexual activity, number of partners; safer sex practices and use condoms; risky practices; past sexually transmitted diseases (STDs) (when treatment, tested for cure); recent exposure to a partner with an STD, hepatitis B, or HIV; other risk factors for hepatitis B or HIV, tested or treated for either of these
Pruritus?	Location (local or diffuse; groin, penis, scrotum, thighs, anus, buttocks); association with a rash, lesions, erythema; use of over-the-counter medications (what brand, provide relief)
Infestations?	Presence of lice, scabies, or fleas; recent exposure; parasites or nits seen; prior treatment (dates, type); overtreatment (e.g., lindane toxicity from overzealous delousing)
Lesions?	Type (macule, papule, ulcer, vesicle, rash, laceration, excoriation), arrangement (single or clustered), location (groin, penis, scrotum, thighs, anus), distribution (symmetrical, asymmetrical, along a dermatome, involving more than one dermatome), associated pain, pruritis, suppuration

Discharge?	Color, character, and amount (scant, profuse; thick, thin; malodorous; clear, white, gray, yellow, green, blood tinged; constant or intermittent) association with urination or ejaculation
Pain?	Type (localized or diffuse); location (groin, penis, scrotum, thighs, anus); history of trauma to the groin or genitals, provocative/palliative factors, quality, region, severity, and timing (see Chapter 1, Table 1–1)
Genitourinary symptoms?	Difficulty initiating stream of urine, change in frequency of urination, urgency, dysuria, hematuria, pyuria, polyuria, oliguria, nocturia, leaking urine, incontinence, or stress incontinence; how long; associated symptoms (fever, malaise, flank pain, abdominal pain, nausea, or vomiting); history of benign prostatic hypertrophy (BPH), prostatitis, renal or urethral calculi
Masses or swelling?	Location (groin, inguinal area, penis, scrotum, thighs, anus); characteristics (tender or nontender; soft or hard; fluctuant or draining) how long has it been there; change in size over time
Infertility?	Past conception; time spent "trying" without success; infertility work-up (patient, partner), results
Sexual dysfunction?	Loss of libido, inability to have an erection, to climax, to ejaculate; premature ejaculation; painful coitus; feelings of ambivalence, insecurity, anxiety, or depression with regard to current relationships
Sexual abuse or assault?	Recent or remote sexual abuse or assault; evaluation and counselling by an experienced crisis team

PHYSICAL EXAMINATION

Equipment

Gloves

Reflex hammer

Materials for genital cultures

Procedures, Techniques, and Findings

1. **Inspect the external genitalia (Fig. 19–1). Assess sexual maturity.**

   Note the distribution of pubic hair (absent in infants and children and thick, extending onto thighs, in adults). Note the shape and size of the penis (usually adult size and shape after puberty). Note size, color, and texture of scrotum (darkened and ruggated after puberty). Assess for sexual maturity (Fig. 19–2).

2. **Inspect and palpate the skin for color, temperature, lesions, masses, excoriations, other lesions, lacerations, abnormalities, infestations, or lack of hygiene.**

   Part the pubic hair as necessary to facilitate thorough examination. Gently move and manipulate the penis and scrotum to allow visualization of their posterior sides. Palpate thoroughly and note the type and location of any noticed lesions (macules, papules, ulcers, vesicles, rash, laceration, excoriation, mass).

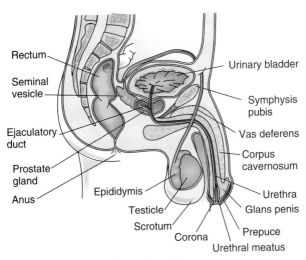

FIGURE 19-1 Anatomy of the male genitalia.

	Pubic hair	Penis	Testes and scrotum
Stage 1 Sexual maturity 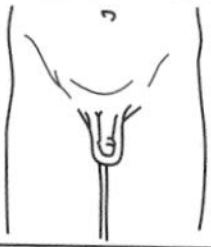	None except for fine body hair as on the abdomen	Size proportional to body size as in childhood	Size proportional to body size as in childhood
Stage 2 Sexual maturity 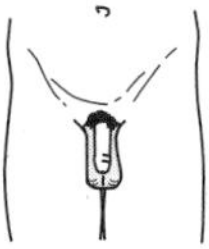	Sparse, long, slightly pigmented, thin hair at the base of the penis	Slight enlargement	Enlargement of testes and scrotum; reddened pigmentation; texture more prominent
Stage 3 Sexual maturity 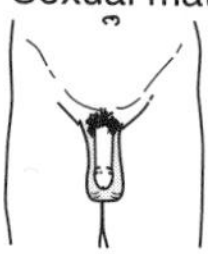	Darkens, becomes more coarse and curly; growth extends over symphysis	Elongation	Enlargement continues
Stage 4 Sexual maturity 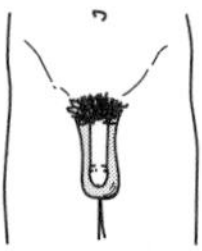	Continues to darken, thicken, and become coarser and more curly	Breadth and length increase; glans develops	Enlargement continues; skin pigmentation darkens
Stage 5 Sexual maturity 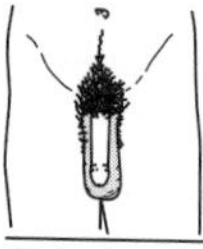	Adult distribution and appearance; growth extends to inner thighs	Adult appearance	Adult appearance
Elderly clients 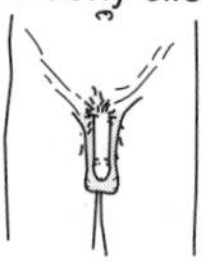	Hair sparse and gray	Decrease in size	Testes hang low in scrotum; scrotum appears pendulous

FIGURE 19-2 Stages of sexual maturity.

3. **Inspect and palpate the prepuce or foreskin in uncircumcised males.**

   Note any lesions, swelling, edema, lacerations, erythema, or ecchymosis. Gently retract the foreskin. Inspect the interior. Pay particular attention to the junction between the prepuce and the glans, as this is often the preferred site of STD-related lesions.

4. **Inspect and palpate the glans.**

   Inspect and palpate the full surface of the glans, noting exact location of any lesions, masses, swelling, edema, abnormalities, erythema, or ecchymosis. The glans will be moist and pink in uncircumcised males, and appear more reddish and dry in circumcised males.

5. **Inspect the urethral meatus for position, abnormalities, and discharge.**

   Note the location of the urinary meatus and check for hypospadias (abnormal position of the meatus, usually on posterior side). Note location and type of lesions or abnormalities. Inspect for prolapse, fissures, and fistulas. Gently compress the glans between your thumb and finger (or allow patient to do this) to open the meatus slightly (Fig. 19–3B). Inspect the color and discharge. Culture any discharge present for gonorrhea, chlamydia, and bacteria. You may also want to do a potassium hydroxide (KOH) and wet prep to look for yeast and trichomonas at this time. (Note: If the patient complains of discharge and none is seen, you may need to milk the shaft of the penis gently to produce a bead of discharge.)

6. **Inspect and palpate the shaft of the penis.**

   Gently manipulate and lift the penis to allow inspection and palpation of the entire surface area. Note exact location and type of lesions, masses, or abnormalities. Palpate for induration and tenderness along the ventral surface (Fig. 19–3A). In infants and children this may be omitted.

7. **Inspect and palpate the scrotum and testes for size, shape, color, temperature, tenderness, lesions, abnormalities.**

   Gently palpate the testicles by grasping them between your thumb and forefinger (Fig. 19–3C). Palpate the epididymis, spermatic cord, and vas deferens. Note any lesions, masses, tenderness, or enlargement. Illuminate the scrotum and testicle if a mass is suspected or an enlargement is observed.

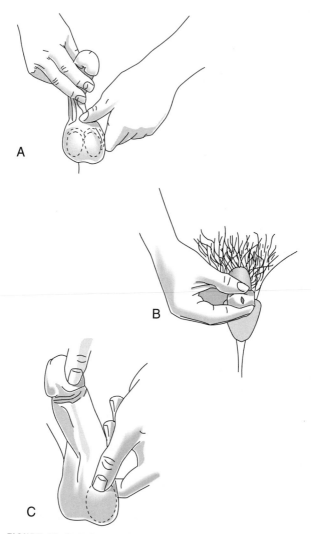

FIGURE 19-3 *A,* Examination of penis and scrotum. *B,* Examination of urethral meatus. *C,* Examination of spermatic cord and testes.

A fluid-filled mass will illuminate well, while a mass filled with blood, pus, or solid tissue will not.

8. **Inspect and palpate for hernias (Fig. 19–4).**

   Ask the patient to stand and bear down as though having a bowel movement. Inspect the inguinal areas and scrotum for any bulging or masses. With one finger, press inward on the loose skin at a low point on the scrotum. Follow the spermatic cord upward by invaginating loose scrotal skin until you can palpate the external inguinal ring. If possible, follow the inguinal canal to the internal inguinal ring. Ask the patient to bear down and again feel for any bulging or masses. If a hernia is palpated, apply gentle pressure and note whether it is reducible. (Never force your finger into the inguinal canal. If you meet with resistance, or the patient complains of pain stop the exam.)

9. **Palpate the prostate gland.**

   See Chapter 20, Assessment of the Anus, Rectum, and Prostate.

NORMAL FINDINGS	ABNORMAL FINDINGS
Skin	
Warm, smooth skin without lesions, ecchymosis, erythema	Hot, red skin indicates cellulitis or inflammation; presence of lesions may indicate dermatitis or venereal disease (macules, secondary syphilis; papules, venereal warts; ulcers, syphilis; vesicles, herpes simplex II; excoriations, lice or scabies; rash, candidiasis)
Pubic hair	
Density of growth and distribution should be consistent with that expected for patient's age group	Abnormal quantity and distribution for age may indicate hormonal imbalances, chronic disease, dermatitis or response to medications; hair loss may be symmetrical and nonscarring, or asymmetrical and scarring

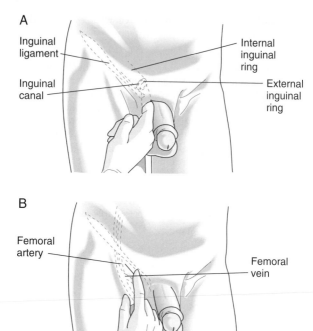

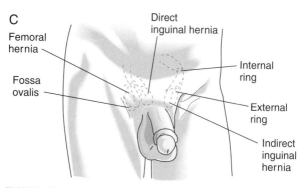

FIGURE 19-4 *A,* Palpation for inguinal hernia. *B,* Palpation for femoral hernia. *C,* Comparative locations of direct inguinal, indirect inguinal, and femoral hernias.

NORMAL FINDINGS	**ABNORMAL FINDINGS**

Prepuce

Normally without lesions, lacerations, edema; easily retractable; smegma, a whitish pasty exudate, may normally be present	Presence of lesions, lacerations, edema, erythema; inability to retract the prepuce (phimosis) or inability to replace a retracted prepuce (paraphimosis) are abnormal and indicate disease

Glans

Appears pink and moist in uncircumcised males, and may appear dry and reddish in circumcised males; no lesions, masses, erythema, ecchymosis	Presence of any lesions or masses as described above; balanitis, or inflammation of the glans with marked erythema; edema

Urethral meatus

A pink, slitlike opening located in the center of the glans; no lesions, masses, or discharge	Hypospadias, or congenital displacement of the urethral meatus (usually on posterior portion of the glans or shaft); urethral prolapse (a perceivable small rosette of prolapsed membranes protruding from the meatus); discharge (clear, yellow, white, or blood-tinged) may indicate urethritis and must be cultured and treated appropriately (Fig. 19–5)

Shaft

No lesions, erythema, ecchymosis, edema	Presence of any lesions as described above may indicate venereal disease; tenderness or induration along the ventral surface may indicate urethral stricture and periurethral inflammation, or carcinoma

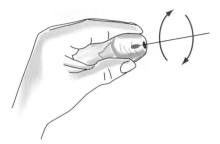

FIGURE 19-5 Culturing genital discharge in the male.

NORMAL FINDINGS	ABNORMAL FINDINGS
Scrotum and testes	

NORMAL FINDINGS	ABNORMAL FINDINGS
Coarse, loose, ruggated skin of slightly darker pigment than the rest of the body; no lesions, erythema, edema, masses, or swelling; sensitive, but not painful, to gentle compression between two fingers; not >1 inch diameter in size; left testis is normally lower than the right	Undescended testes; cryptorchidism or poorly developed scrotum on one or both sides; presence of lesions, masses, edema, erythema, ecchymosis

Nontender swelling or mass:

Hydrocele/spermatocele: fluid-filled cysts of the tunica vaginalis and epididymis that transilluminate

Testicular cancer: a hard, palpable nodule usually on anterior side of the testis

Tender swelling or mass:

Scrotal edema: from chronic exacerbated congestive heart failure, chronic renal failure, or nephrotic syndrome

Epididymitis: acute bacterial infection of epididymis. May be accompanied by urethritis and discharge

Testicular torsion: occasionally torsion of

Vas deferens and spermatic cord

No masses, thickening, or tenderness	Any swelling, mass, or tenderness
	Varicocele: beadlike nodules or varicosities (bag of worms) palpated usually on the left side
	Thickening of the vas deferens or spermatic cord may occur with chronic infections and tuberculosis

Hernias

None	Direct inguinal hernia: palpated above the inguinal ligament close to the external inguinal ring; it bulges anteriorly, does not travel down the inguinal canal, and may, but rarely does, invade the scrotum
	Indirect inguinal hernia: palpated above the inguinal ligament close to the internal inguinal ring; it travels down the inguinal canal and often invades the scrotum
	Femoral hernia: palpated below the inguinal ligament and appears more lateral than inguinal hernias; difficult to distinguish from enlarged inguinal lymph nodes
	All hernias may become painful if strangulation occurs, either by torsion of bowel or compression by surrounding tissue.

Clinical Notes

Palpate external genitalia gently so as not to cause the patient undue embarrassment by stimulating an erection.

Never force your finger into the inguinal canal. If you are met with firm resistance or the patient complains of pain, stop the examination.

Testicular torsion is a surgical emergency. If suspected, the patient must receive immediate attention to prevent the necrosis of a testis.

Patients should be instructed in the techniques of testicular self-examination.

 Geriatric Considerations

	NORMAL FINDINGS:
Pubic hair	Thin, sparse, gray
Testes	Less firm, smaller in size, skin less taut, resulting in a more pendulous appearance
Penis	Decrease in size

Penile epispadias

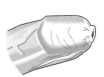

Phimois

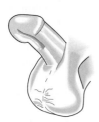

Penile hypospadias

Paraphimosis

FIGURE 19-6 Abnormalities of male genitalia.

Text continued on page 342

TABLE 19-1 Common Abnormalities of the Male Genitalia

Abnormality	Definition/Causation	Basis for Diagnosis
Hydrocele	An accumulation of serous fluid between the visceral and parietal layers of the tunica vaginalis	Transilluminates; fingers can get above the mass
Scrotal hernia	A hernia within the scrotum	Bowel sounds auscultated; does not transilluminate; fingers cannot get above the mass
Varicocele	Abnormal dilatation and tortuosity of the veins of the pampiniform plexus; often described as a "bag of worms" in the scrotum	Complaints of a dragging sensation or dull pain in the scrotal area; feels like a soft bag of worms; collapses when the scrotum is elevated and increases when the scrotum is dependent; more commonly appears on the left side; usually appears at puberty

Table continued on following page

TABLE 19-1 Common Abnormalities of the Male Genitalia *Continued*

Abnormality	Definition/Causation	Basis for Diagnosis
Spermatocele	An epididymal cyst resulting from a partial obstruction of the spermatic tubules	Transilluminates; round mass, feels like a third testis; painless
Tuberculosis	May be a result of benign or malignant neoplasms, syphilis, or tuberculosis	Nodules are not tender; in tuberculosis lesions, vas deferens often feels beaded
Epididymitis	An inflammation of the epididymis, usually resulting from *Escherichia coli, Neisseria gonorrhoeae,* or *Mycobacterium tuberculosis* organisms	Spermatic cord often thickened and indurated; pain relieved by elevation

TABLE 19-1	Common Abnormalities of the Male Genitalia *Continued*	
Abnormality	Definition/Causation	Basis for Diagnosis
Torsion of the spermatic cord	Axial rotation or volvulus of the spermatic cord, resulting in infarction of the testicle	Elevated mass; pain not relieved by further elevation; more common in childhood or adolescence; history of extreme pain and tenderness of the testis, followed by hyperemic swelling and hydrocele
Testicular tumor	Multiple causes	Usually not painful; hydroceles may develop as a result of a tumor— if a testis cannot be palpated, fluid needs to be aspirated so that the testes can be accurately evaluated

Clinical Notes

Size changes do not mean a change in libido or function. Most older men remain sexually active.

 Pediatric Considerations

History

Masturbatory behaviors?

Known sexual abuse?

Development of secondary sexual characteristics?

Sexually active? Known to family or confidential?

Knowledge base re: contraception and STDs?

Conflicts re: sexual identity/orientation?

NORMAL FINDINGS	ABNORMAL FINDINGS (FIG. 19–6, TABLE 19–1)
Newborn and infant	
Foreskin adheres to glans penis	
Edema, bruising of the genitals postdelivery	Hypospadias: meatus located along ventral surface of glans or shaft of penis; foreskin incomplete
Testes in scrotum	
Testes in inguinal canal, can be milked down into scrotum	Undescended testicle
Hydrocele: scrotum transilluminates	
	Hernias: inguinal or scrotal mass
Child	

Foreskin retractable

Clinical Notes

Refer to Figure 19–2 to determine degree of sexual maturation.

Assessment of the Anus, Rectum, and Prostate

HISTORY AND CURRENT STATUS QUESTIONS

Pruritus?	Area, date of onset, associated rash; lice, scabies, or pinworms. Does itch occur at any particular time of day? Is it associated with particular food or medication
Lesions?	Type (macules, papules, ulcers, vesicles, excoriations, lacerations), location, length of time present, tender or nontender, exudate, obstruction of the anus, interference with normal defecation and hygiene
Abdominal distention or mass?	Internal or external hemorrhoids, prolapsed rectum, rectal mass or cancer, perianal abscess, palpable or enlarged inguinal nodes, distention of the abdomen or palpable abdominal masses (evidence of obstruction or urinary retention)
Flatulence?	Diet high in gas-producing foods (onions, cabbage, carbonated drinks)
Diet?	Diet high in fat or low in fiber
Bowel habits?	Diarrhea, constipation, urgency, frequency, nocturnal defecation, incontinence of stool, blood or mucus in the stool; characteristics of stool brown, yellow, gray, black; watery, loose, formed, greasy, hard; pencil, ribbon, or pipe-stemmed stool

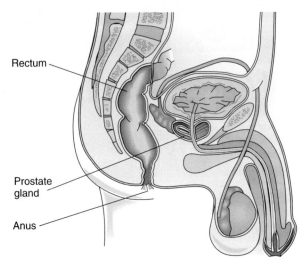

FIGURE 20-1 Anal canal, rectum, and prostate.

Genitourinary symptoms?	Difficulty initiating a stream of urine, change in frequency of urination, urgency, dysuria, hematuria, pyuria, polyuria, oliguria, nocturia, leaking urine, stress incontinence, or incontinence; duration of symptoms; associated symptoms (fever, malaise, flank pain, abdominal pain, nausea, or vomiting); history of benign prostatic hypertrophy (BPH), prostatitis, renal or ureteral calculi
Pain?	Palliative/provocative factors, quality, region, severity, timing (PQRST) type (low back, low abdominal, rectal, anal) association with defecation (concomitant, increase)

PHYSICAL EXAMINATION

Equipment

Gloves

Hemoccult card test solution

Procedures, Techniques, and Findings

1. **Inspect and palpate perianal tissue and perineum.**

   If the rectal exam is to be performed at the end of a gyn exam, the patient may remain in the semirecumbent or lithotomy position; otherwise, position the patient (male or female) on the side in the Sims position with knees slightly flexed. Gently retract the buttocks with your gloved hands, and inspect the anal and perianal tissue. Note color, texture, lesions, masses, prolapse, hemmorrhoids, skin breakdown, etc.

2. **Inspect for the appearance of protrusions or masses with straining.**

   Ask the patient to bear down as though attempting a bowel movement. Inspect for protrusions or masses, including prolapse, polyps, and hemmorrhoids.

3. **Perform a digital exam to palpate the anus, rectum, and prostate.**

   Press gently against the anal sphincter with the gloved and lubricated index fingerpad. Ask patient to bear down and gently press fingertip into the opening of the anus (Fig. 20–2A).

4. **Assess the tone and musculature of the anal sphincter.**

   Palpate the entire surface of the anal sphincter. Ask the patient to tighten the buttocks around your finger to allow assessment of tone and strength of the sphincter.

5. **Palpate the muscular anal ring and rectum.**

   Palpate the entire surface of the muscular anal ring by turning the finger in a circular motion around its own axis. Move further inward to the rectum and repeat. Note any palpable lesions, masses, lacerations, or other abnormalities (Fig. 20–2B).

6. **Palpate for high masses.**

   With finger as far into the rectum as possible, ask the patient to bear down. Feel for any descending masses.

7. **Palpate prostate in men.**

   Turn your finger to palpate the anterior rectal wall. Gently palpate the prostate. Try to identify the two lateral lobes and

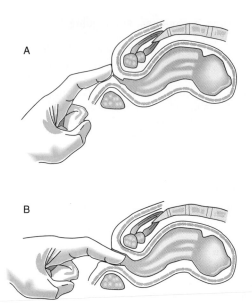

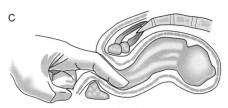

FIGURE 20-2 Assessment of the rectum and prostate. *A,* Entering the anal opening. *B,* Examining the rectum. *C,* Examining the prostate.

the median sulcus. Note any enlargement, irregularity in shape, palpable mass, tenderness, or softening (bogginess) (Fig. 20–2C).

8. Palpate the uterus and cervix in women.

Turn your finger to palpate the anterior rectal wall. Gently palpate the uterus and cervix. Note any enlargement, irregularity in shape, palpable mass, tenderness, or softening (bogginess).

9. **Examine fecal material.**

Withdraw your gloved finger and examine the fecal material on the glove for color (brown, gray, yellow, black) and consistency (watery, loose, greasy, formed, hard). Using a Hemoccult card (Fig. 20–3) test the stool for occult blood.

NORMAL FINDINGS	ABNORMAL FINDINGS
Perianal tissue	
No lesions, masses, erythema, or skin breakdown; tissue may appear slightly darker in pigmentation	Fecal matter or other signs of poor hygiene, erythema, ecchymosis, skin breakdown, fistula openings, sinus tracts, abscesses, masses, or lesions
Anus	
Slightly reddened and closed; no lesions, masses, protrusions, hemorrhoids; urge to defecate may occur when finger is inserted; sphincter will normally tighten snuggly around finger.	Erythema, ecchymosis, edema, skin breakdown, decubitus ulcer, rectal prolapse (rosette), hemorrhoids, polyps, protrusions, lesions, masses, lacerations, fissures, fistulas, sinus tracts, and poor sphincter tone
Rectum	
Smooth, without masses, lesions, tenderness	Tenderness, lesions, masses, palpable rectal shelf (often secondary to peritoneal metastatic tissue); presence of a "high mass" descending against fingertip when the patient bears down

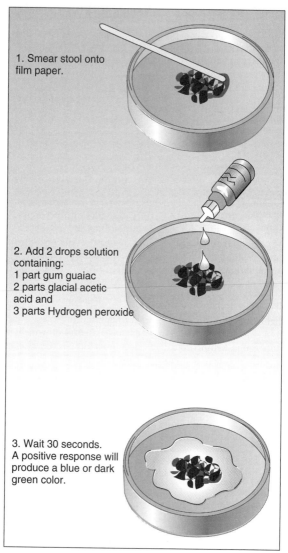

FIGURE 20-3 Guaiac testing of stool.

NORMAL FINDINGS	ABNORMAL FINDINGS

Prostate

Palpable only after onset of puberty; normally not >1 cm protruding into rectum; rubbery and smooth to palpation; two lateral lobes and median sulcus may be distinguishable; should be nontender, without palpable masses	Protrusion into rectum of >1 cm; enlarged, nodular, or irregular in shape; boggy or tender on palpation; any hard palpable mass

Uterus and cervix

Rubbery, smooth, and nontender	Any enlargement, irregularity of surface, palpable mass, or tenderness

Fecal material

Normally formed, brown stool, without frank or occult blood	Yellow, gray, or black stool; watery, loose, hard, or impacted stool; frank or occult blood (guaiac or Hemoccult test required)

Clinical Notes

Occasionally patients present with a foreign object in the rectum as their chief complaint. Digital examination should be done carefully so as not to push the object further down into the rectum.

If a Hemoccult test is positive, the patient should be referred for further testing to rule out colorectal malignancy.

Sexual assault or abuse must be considered whenever anal bruising or lacerations are observed.

 ## Geriatric Considerations

	NORMAL FINDINGS
Rectum	Relaxation of the internal sphincter inhibited
Prostate	Enlarged

Clinical Notes

Difficulty starting and stopping the urine stream can be the result of an enlarged prostate. Obtain a clear picture of voiding patterns.

 Pediatric Considerations

History

Stool pattern

NORMAL FINDINGS	ABNORMAL FINDINGS
Newborn	
Anus	
Patent anus	
Tight rectal sphincter	Imperforate anus
	Meconium ileus
Passes meconium stool within 24 hours	
	Pencil-thin stools

Assessment of the Musculoskeletal System

HISTORY AND CURRENT STATUS QUESTIONS

Personal history of musculoskeletal disease

History of arthritis, joint disease, collagen vascular disease, or cancer; illness affecting the strength or function of any muscle groups; recent or remote trauma (part of the body affected; resultant amputations, fractures, crushed, torn, or mangled muscles; orthopaedic or arthroscopic surgery); occupational or recreational activity likely to inflict a particular overuse injury

Family history of musculoskeletal disease

History of family members with rheumatoid arthritis, gout, osteoarthritis, lupus, sickle cell disease, congenital deformities of the bones or muscles, progressive myositis, multiple sclerosis, muscular dystrophy, myasthenia gravis, polio, or cancer (relation of the family member to the patient, age of onset of the illness, and if the family member is deceased, illness or condition responsible for death)

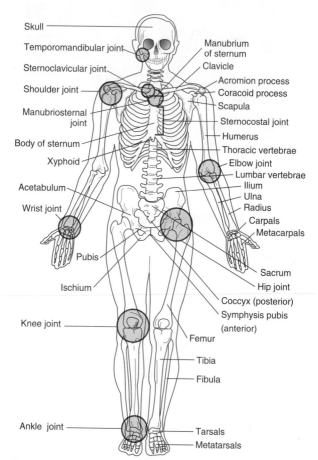

FIGURE 21-1 Bones and joints.

Pain?

Provocative/palliative factors, quality, region (joint, muscle), severity, and timing (at rest, with exercise, a considerable time after exertion, upon awakening, or with extreme temperature or weather changes (PQRST; see Table 1–1)

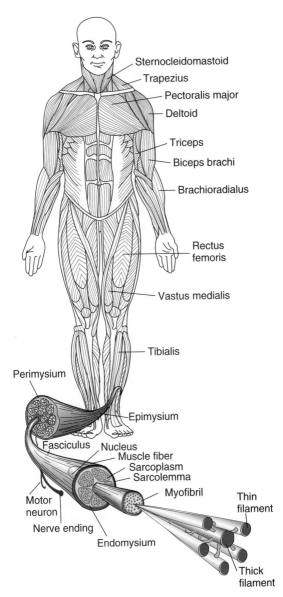

FIGURE 21-2 Muscles and motor unit.

Change in range of motion (ROM)?	Limited ability to move a particular joint, inability to bend at the waist, reach, grasp, hold, lift, stretch, walk, run, turn the head, sit, stand, or lie down as previously able
Change in size of an extremity or swelling of a joint?	Insidious or acute onset; associated edema, erythema, ecchymosis, pain, or heat of the affected area; trauma
Erythema?	Does the patient complain of erythema or areas of reddened skin surrounding a joint or extremity?
Temperature?	Fever (measured with a thermometer; oral or rectally), highest temperature recorded; joints, surrounding tissues, or extremities hot to the touch
Crepitus?	Unusual creaking or cracking sounds whenever a joint is moved or palpated
Deformity?	Malalignment, new or poorly healed fracture, arthritic nodule, tumor, or abnormal curvature (as in the spine)
Loss of height?	Osteoporosis in elderly (more often women) if unrelated to surgical procedures; severe kyphosis (hunched back) or compression fractures of the spine
Muscle weakness?	Muscles affected, characteristics (unilateral or bilateral, constant or intermittent, insidious or acute onset), associated with any trauma or surgery, effect on ADL

TABLE 21–1	Classification of Joints	
Type of Joint	**Example**	**Description**
Synarthrosis		*No movement is permitted*
Suture	Cranial sutures	United by thin layer of fibrous tissue
Synchondrosis	Joint between the epiphysis and diaphysis of long bones	A temporary joint in which the cartilage is replaced by bone later in life
Amphiarthrosis		Slightly *movable joint*
Symphysis	Symphysis pubis	Bones are connected by a fibrocartilage disk
Syndesmosis	Radius–ulna articulation	Bones are connected by ligaments
Diarthrosis (synovial)		*Freely movable*
		Enclosed by joint capsule, lined with synovial membrane
Ball and socket	Hip	Widest range of motion, movement in all planes
Hinge	Elbow	Motion limited to flexion and extension in a single plane
Pivot	Atlantoaxis	Motion limited to rotation
Condyloid	Wrist between radius and carpals	Motion in two planes at right angles to each other, but no radial rotation
Saddle	Thumb at carpometacarpal joint	Motion in two planes at right angles to each other, but no axial rotation
Gliding	Intervertebral	Motion limited to gliding

PHYSICAL EXAMINATION

Equipment

Tape measure

Goniometer

Procedures, Techniques, and Findings

1. **Assess the patient's posture, stance, and gait.**

   Observe the patient's posture, stance, and gait, inconspicuously as he/she enters the examining room.

TABLE 21-2	Muscle Function Terminology
Term	**Definition and Example**
Abduction	Lateral movement of a body part away from the midline of the body. *Example: The arm is abducted when it is moved away from the body.*
Adduction	Lateral movement of a body part toward the midline of the body. *Example: The arm is moved from an outstretched position to a position alongside the body.*
Circumduction	Movement of the distal part of the limb to trace a complete circle while the proximal end of the bone remains fixed. *Example: The leg is outstretched and moved in a circle.*
Flexion	The state of being bent.
Extension	The state of being in a straight line.
Hyperextension	The state of exaggerated extension. It often results in an angle >180 degrees. *Example: The spine is hyperextended when looking overhead, toward the ceiling.*
Dorsiflexion	Backward bending of the hand or foot. *Example: The foot is in dorsiflexion when the toes are brought up as though to point them at the knee.*
Plantar flexion	Flexion of the foot. *Example: The foot is in plantar flexion in the footdrop position.*
Rotation	Turning on an axis; the turning of a body part on the axis provided by its joint. *Example: A thumb is rotated when it is moved to make a circle.*
Internal rotation	A body part turning on its axis toward the midline of the body. *Example: A leg is rotated internally when it turns inward at the hip and the toes point toward the midline of the body.*
External rotation	A body part turning on its axis away from the midline of the body. *Example: A leg is rotated externally when it turns outward at the hip and the toes point away from the midline of the body.*
Special Movements	
Pronation	The assumption of the prone position. *Example: Lying flat on the abdomen*
Supination	The assumption of the supine position. *Example: Lying flat on the back*
Inversion	Movement of the sole of the foot inward (occurs at the ankle)
Eversion	Movement of the sole of the foot outward (occurs at the ankle)

2. **Prepare the patient for the examination.**

   Ask the patient to undress to his/her underwear. Instruct the patient to stand, sit, or lie down as necessary through the course of the examination.

3. **Inspect for any gross abnormalities.**

   Note any gross, or obvious abnormalities that are easily noticed on an initial glancing head to toe inspection (i.e., amputations, congenital deformities of extremities, contractures, paralysis, etc.).

4. **Inspect and palpate the skin and surrounding tissue of all bones, joints and muscle groups to be examined.**

   Refer to Chapter 6, Assessment of the Skin, Hair, and Nails.

5. **Inspect and palpate the temporomandibular joint (TMJ) and jaw**

   Inspect and palpate for abnormalities, deformities, masses, tenderness, or asymmetry. Place two or three fingertips of each hand over the TMJ joints simultaneously. Ask the patient to open widely and close the mouth two or three times. Palpate for any unusual clicking sounds, sliding, or "catching" of the joint (Fig. 21–3). With the patient's mouth open as wide as possible, attempt to vertically insert three fingers held side by side between the upper and lower teeth. Ask the patient to slide the lower jaw forward and from side to side, so that the lower teeth protrude beyond and over lap the upper teeth in each instance.

6. **Inspect and palpate the neck and spine.**

   Inspect and palpate the neck and cervical spine. Then inspect and palpate the full length of the spine with the patient standing erect and again with the patient bending over at the waist. Observe the spinal curvature from directly behind the patient, and again from a side view. Normally the cervical spine is concave, the thoracic spine convex, and the lumbar spine concave. Note any abnormal curvatures of the spine, palpable masses, tenderness, or irregularities of alignment.

7. **Assess the ROM of the neck (Fig. 21–4).**

   Flexion: touch chin to chest.

   Hyperextension: bend head backward with chin pointing toward ceiling.

   Text continued on page 360

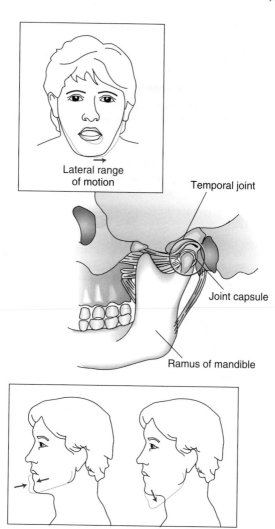

FIGURE 21-3 Range of motion: temporal mandibular joint and jaw.

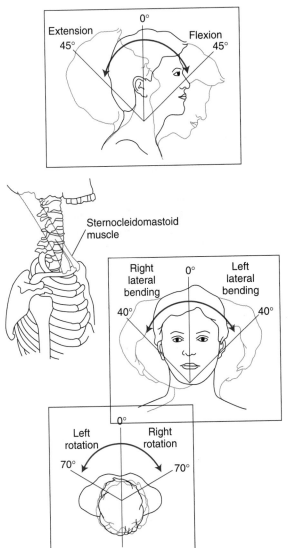

FIGURE 21–4 Range of motion: neck.

Rotation: turn head to the left and right with ears facing the back and chest.

Lateral bending: bend head laterally with ear toward shoulder.

8. **Assess the ROM of the spine (Fig. 21–5).**

   Flexion: bend forward at the waist.

   Extension: bend backward at the waist.

   Rotation: with feet planted and toes pointing forward, rotate the torso so that the shoulders attempt to face forward and backward.

   Lateral bending: bend laterally at the waist with shoulders toward feet.

9. **Inspect and palpate the upper and lower extremities, assessing each joint and associated muscle groups for:**

   Work your way down from top to bottom, assessing first the right and then the left side. Begin with the shoulders. Assess the right and then the left shoulder, the right and then the left elbow, etc., moving down through the wrists, fingers, hips, knees, ankles, and toes.

   Condition of skin and surrounding tissue

   Inspect the skin and surrounding tissue for erythema, swelling, edema, masses, and lesions. Palpate for temperature, tenderness, crepitus (abnormal sounds), masses, or bony abnormalities.

   Contralateral symmetry

   Assess contralateral symmetry. Note any difference in size, shape, position, or alignment of like joints.

   Muscle tone and strength

   Muscle tone and strength may be assessed at the same time as ROM. Assess muscle tone by noting the degree of resistance felt on passive range of motion. Normally a slight resistance will be felt. Assess muscle strength by asking the patient to pull away from or push against an opposing force that you impose. Repeat the same maneuver with the contralateral joint and assess bilateral muscle strength.

   Stability of joint

   Assess the stability of each joint. In general, grasp and stabilize the joint on the proximal side with one hand

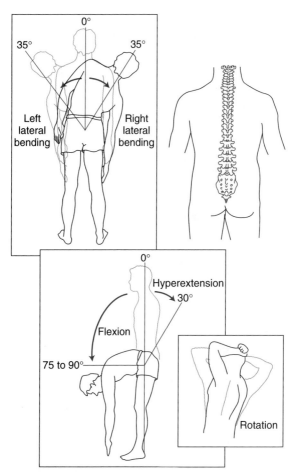

FIGURE 21-5 Range of motion: spine.

while attempting to move the joint with the other hand from the distal end. Note any abnormal movements, crepitus, unusual sounds, abnormal ROM, or tenderness associated with these maneuvers. To further differentiate suspected tendon or ligament damage, refer to the special maneuvers described for each specific joint.

Range of motion

Put each joint through full passive range of motion (as detailed below). Note the angle at which the joint is freely able to bend in each position. Compare the ROM of contralateral joints. For greater accuracy measure the joint angles with a goniometer (Fig. 21–6).

10. **Shoulders**

Range of motion (Fig. 21–7)

Flexion: lift arm forward and above head with arm straight.

Horizontal flexion: abduct arm straight and horizontal to the floor, then move arm backward toward the spine.

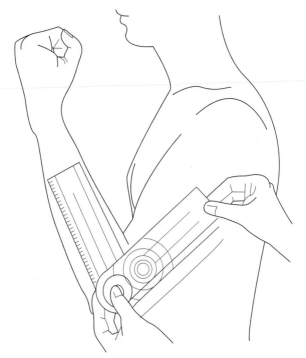

FIGURE 21-6 Use of the goniometer.

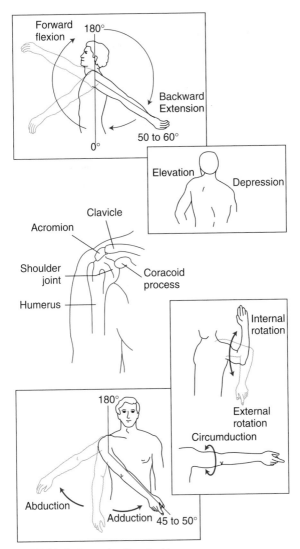

FIGURE 21-7 Range of motion: shoulders.

Extension: move arm backward with arm straight.

Horizontal extension: abduct arm horizontal to floor and then bring arm across chest.

Abduction: lift arm straight up above head.

Adduction: adduct arm toward midline of trunk.

Special maneuvers

11. **Elbows**

Range of motion (Fig. 21–8)

Flexion: bend lower arm up toward biceps.

Extension: Open arm to resting fully extended position.

Hyperextension: extend arm beyond normal resting position.

Supination: turn lower arm so that front faces upward.

Pronation: turn lower arm so that front faces downward.

Special maneuvers

12. **Wrists**

Range of motion (Fig. 21–9)

Flexion: flex wrist toward lower arm.

Extension: extend wrist backward.

Radial deviation: deviate wrist toward radius.

Ulnar deviation: deviate wrist toward ulna.

Special maneuvers

13. **Fingers**

Range of motion (Fig. 21–10)

Flexion: close fingers into a fist.

Extension: fully open fingers.

Abduction: spread fingers apart.

Adduction: cross fingers together so that they touch and overlap.

Opposition: touch each finger with the thumb of the same hand.

Special maneuvers

14. **Hips**

Range of motion (Fig. 21–11)

Text continued on page 369

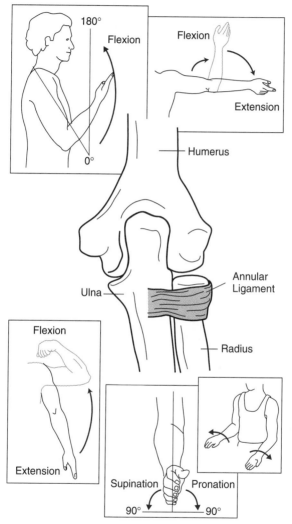

FIGURE 21-8 Range of motion: elbows.

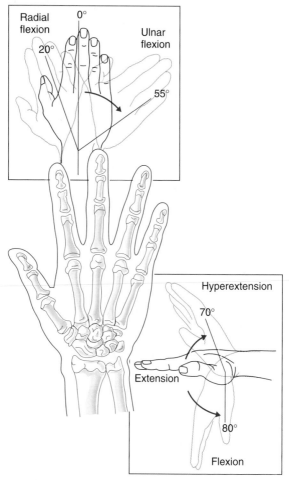

FIGURE 21-9   Range of motion: wrists.

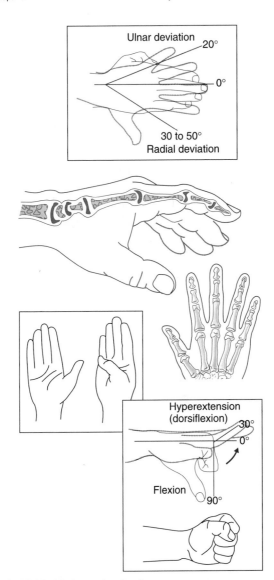

FIGURE 21-10 Range of motion: fingers.

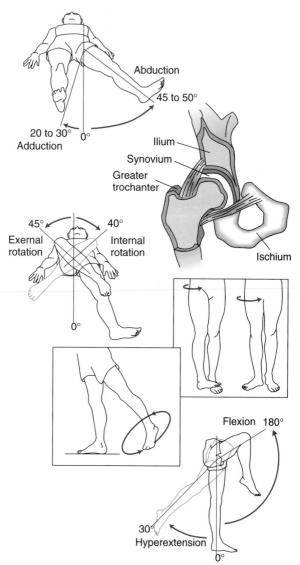

FIGURE 21-11 Range of motion: hips.

Flexion with straight knee: raise leg straight up without bending the knee.

Flexion with knee bent: raise leg straight up with knee bent.

Extension: lie prone and extend leg backward.

Abduction: abduct partially flexed leg outward.

Adduction: adduct partially flexed leg inward.

Internal rotation: flex knee and swing foot away from midline.

External rotation: flex knee and swing foot toward midline.

Special maneuvers

15. **Knees**

Range of motion (Fig. 21–12)

Flexion: Fully bend knee with calf touching thigh.

Hyperextension: extend knee beyond normal point of extension.

Internal rotation: rotate knee and lower leg toward midline.

Special maneuvers

16. **Ankles**

Range of motion (Fig. 21–13)

Dorsiflexion: bend dorsal part of foot upward with toes pointing toward head.

Plantar flexion: bend foot downward with toes pointing downward.

Eversion: turn foot away from midline.

Inversion: turn foot toward midline.

Special maneuvers

17. **Toes**

Range of motion (Fig. 21–14)

Flexion: curl toes under foot.

Extension: lift toes to point upward.

Abduction: spread toes apart.

Adduction: normally unable.

Special maneuvers

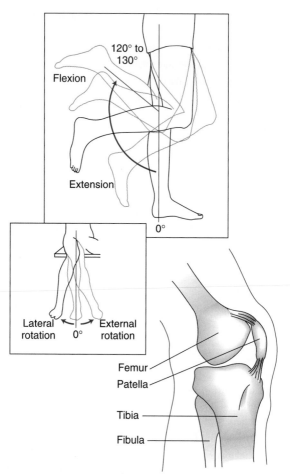

FIGURE 21-12 Range of motion: knees.

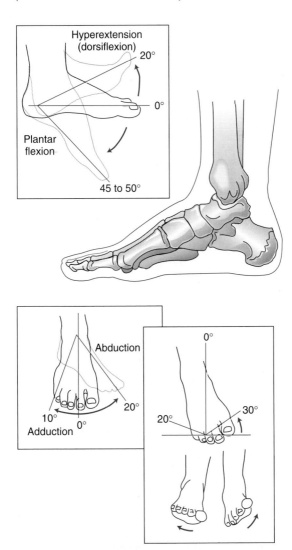

FIGURE 21-13 Range of motion: ankles.

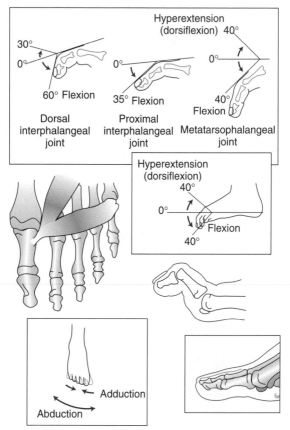

FIGURE 21-14 Range of motion: toes.

NORMAL FINDINGS	ABNORMAL FINDINGS
Posture	
Ability to stand erect, with head up, face forward, arms hanging straight at the sides, shoulders and hips parallel, legs straight with both knees	Inability to stand erect, exhibiting hunched, bent, stooped posture; abnormal curvature of the spine, as in kyphosis (accentuated

and feet side by side and a few inches apart; contralateral extremities equal in size, shape, and length, and symmetrical

lordosis) or scoliosis (lateral bending of the spine) (Fig. 21–15); contractures or deformities of the extremities

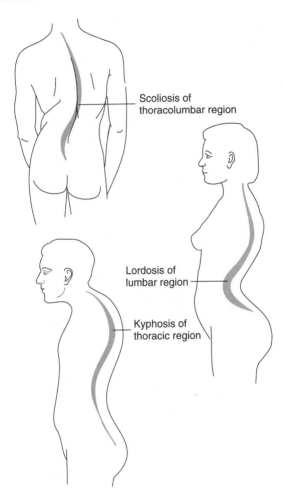

Scoliosis of
thoracolumbar region

Lordosis of
lumbar region

Kyphosis of
thoracic region

FIGURE 21-15 Abnormalities of the spine.

NORMAL FINDINGS	ABNORMAL FINDINGS
Stance	
Ability to stand comfortably without assistance or extrinsic support and without swaying or loss of balance on both feet or on one foot at a time; both feet firmly planted a few inches apart with toes and heels on the ground; toes pointing forward and the weight evenly distributed on both feet	Inability to stand either on two feet or on one foot without assistance or support; evidence of uneven distribution of weight: swaying, stumbling, or loss of balance, favoring one foot, standing on the heels, toes, or edges of the feet, uneven depths of footprints, etc.; toes pointing either laterally or medially rather than straight ahead
Gait	
Ability to walk with equal and symmetrical strides with respect to timing, weight bearing, and distance; steps consisting of a rhythmic planting of first the heel and then the toe of the foot; toes consistently pointing forward; slight swaying back and forth while walking, but no unsteadiness or loss of balance	Evidence of an unsteady gait, excessive swaying, loss of balance, shuffling, limping, propulsive, veering in one direction, exhibiting foot drop or foot lag or any irregularity in the timing of the stride
Skin	
Color Slightly darker in areas most often exposed to sunlight and lighter in areas usually clothed (refer to Chapter 6, Assessment of the Skin, Hair, and Nails)	Hyper or hypopigmentation, erythema, ecchymosis, pale, ashen, gray, or cyanotic; redness suggests gouty arthritis, septic arthritis, or rheumatic fever
Lesions No lesions, masses, lacerations, scars	Presence of macules, papules, vesicles, ulcers, lacerations, scars, masses, or

other lesions; subcutaneous
nodules may be present in
rheumatoid arthritis and
rheumatic fever

Swelling or edema
No swelling or edema

Swelling, edema (pitting or
nonpitting) (see Fig. 16–5)
or palpable effusion of an
underlying joint

Skinfolds
Symmetrical in number and
size over contralateral extremities

Asymmetry of contralateral
skinfolds may suggest malalignment of a bone or joint
(fracture or dislocation)

Temperature
Warm, not hot to touch

Hot to touch, tactile fever;
"hot joint" may represent
gouty arthritis, septic arthritis, rheumatic fever, cellulitis, or a localized infection in
the skin or subcutaneous
tissue

Muscles

Contralateral symmetry
Contralateral muscle groups
symmetrical in size, shape,
contour, and position; tone
and strength may vary normally, with increased tone
and strength demonstrated
on the dominant side

Asymmetry in size, shape,
contour, diameter, position;
Wide variance in tone or
strength between contralateral muscle groups

Tone
A particular muscle or
muscle group will have
normal tone if slight resistance is demonstrated
against passive ROM

Hypertonic muscle exhibits
increased resistance to
passive ROM; hypotonic
muscle presents as boggy, fat,
flabby or flaccid muscle that
offers little or no resistance
against passive ROM

TABLE 21-3	Scale for Muscle Strength
Scale	
0	No muscular contraction
1	Barely flicker of contraction
2	Active movement with gravity removed
3	Active movement against gravity
4	Active movement against gravity and some resistance
5	Active movement against full resistance with no fatigue

Normal strength ranges from 3 to 5.

Adapted from Bales B: A Guide to Physical Examination and History Taking, 5th ed., p. 526. Philadelphia: JB Lippincott, 1991.

NORMAL FINDINGS

Strength
Capable of providing significant resistance to the opposing force imposed; this resistance (or strength) should be relatively equal when compared to the contralateral muscle or muscle group; dominant hand and arm may normally be slightly stronger; normal muscle strength should range between 3 and 5, as described in Bates' assessment of muscle strength scale (Table 21–3)

Bones and joints

Contralateral symmetry
Contralateral bones and joints should be symmetrical in size, shape, position, alignment, stability, and ROM

Change in size or shape
Contralateral bones and joints equal in size and shape

ABNORMAL FINDINGS

Measure the size and circumference of any muscle or muscle groups that demonstrate weakness (or range from 0 to 2 on Bates' scale); smaller circumference and size of a particular muscle or muscle group may indicate atrophy; conversely, an unusually large muscle may indicate hypertrophy

Asymmetry secondary to congenital abnormalities, arthritis, bony tumor, fractures, dislocations, adhesions, or surgery

Position and alignment

Normally positioned and well aligned

Malalignment secondary to fracture, dislocation, congenital anomalies, or surgical procedures

Stability

No abnormal movements, ROM, or sounds upon movement of joints or use of special maneuvers

Instability of a joint without associated dislocation usually indicates tendon or ligament damage

ROM

Ability to move joints passively in all directions and degrees usual for the specific joints, as further described below

Inability or limited ability of a joint to passively move through ROM maneuvers because of stiffness or pain

Jaw (TMJ)

Ability to open and close the jaw freely without pain, clicking, or abnormal sounds, to admit three fingers held together and perpendicular to upper and lower teeth, and to move lower jaw forward so that the bottom teeth overlap the top teeth, and side to side so that the bottom side teeth overlap the top side teeth

Abnormal clicking sound when opening and closing the jaw; malalignment of the upper and lower jaw; inability to move lower jaw sideways or forward; lockjaw (inability to open or close mouth); pain on mastication or movement of the jaw

Neck

Concave curvature of the neck or cervical spine when viewed from the side; no palpable pain or masses

Normal ROM

    Flexion: 70 to 90 degrees

    Hyperextension: 55 degrees

    Rotation: 70 degrees

    Lateral bending: 35 degrees

Pain, palpable masses, compression fractures, lesions, masses, or abnormal curvature; tight palpable cordlike trapezius muscle suggests muscle spasm; chronic pain may be secondary to postural strain; acute recurrent neck pain may be secondary to a herniated intervertebral disc pressing on a nerve root, or cervical spondylosis (degenerative joint disease of one or

NORMAL FINDINGS	ABNORMAL FINDINGS
	more discs in the cervical spine with narrowing of the disc spaces and presence of bony spurs)

Spine
Convex thoracic spine and concave lumbar sacral spine when viewed from the side; no abnormal lateral curvatures; no palpable masses, pain, compression fractures
Normal ROM
    Flexion: 75 degrees
    Extension: 30 degrees
    Rotation: 30 degrees
    Lateral bending: 35 degrees
	Abnormal curvature of the spine, including kyphosis (an accentuated posterior curvature of the thoracic spine, lordosis), sway-back (an accentuated lumbar curvature), scoliosis (a lateral curvature of the spine), and ankylosing spondylitis (evidenced by the persistence of the lumbar concavity and failure of the spinous processes to separate when the patient bends over at the waist); a herniated disc may be tender on palpation; spondylolisthesis (a forward slipping and fusing of the vertebra) may be palpable

Shoulder
Ability to move freely on passive range of motion; no swelling, ecchymosis, lesions, or tenderness; no fractures or dislocation; shoulders symmetrical in size, shape, contour, muscle tone and strength, and ROM
Normal ROM:
    Flexion: 180 degrees
    Horizontal flexion: 130 degrees
    Extension: 60 degrees
	Pain secondary to arthritis, inflammation, infection, bursitis, tendonitis, bony spurs, calcific deposits, masses, fractures, or dislocations; frozen shoulder (inability to abduct the arm without characteristic "shrugging") suggests a rupture of the supraspinatous tendon or rotator cuff injury

Horizontal extension:
45 degrees

Abduction: 180 degrees

Adduction: 45 degrees

Elbow

Normal ROM:

Flexion: 150 degrees

Extension:
150 degrees

Hyperextension: 0 to
10 degrees

Supination:
90 degrees

Pronation:
90 degrees

Wrist

Normal ROM:

Flexion: 80 to 90 degrees

Extension: 70 degrees

Radial deviation:
20 degrees

Ulnar deviation: 30 to
50 degrees

Fingers

Normal ROM:

Flexion: 80 to 100 degrees
(depends on specific joint)

Extension: 0 to 45 degrees
(depending on specific
joint)

Subcutaneous nodules on
the extensor surface of the
ulna suggest rheumatoid
arthritis; a tender lateral
epicondyle suggests tennis
elbow; swelling, inflammation, or thickening of the
olecranon gooves suggests
olecranon arthritis or bursitis

Ganglion cyst (a cystic
round, nontender swelling
along the tendon sheaths or
joint capsules on the dorsum
of the hand or wrists that
becomes more prominent
when the wrist is flexed and
obscured when the wrist is
extended), carpal tunnel
syndrome (compression of
the median nerve that produces numbness and tingling
over the palmar surface of
the thumb, index, middle,
and part of the ring finger,
gonococcal arthritis: (unilateral tenderness of wrist; may
be hot and erythematous)

Arthritic nodules and deformities; atrophy of the thenar
eminence may indicate
median nerve damage;
atrophy of the hypothenar
space may indicate ulnar

NORMAL FINDINGS

Abduction: 20 degrees

Adduction: able to cross fingers together so that they touch and overlap

Opposition: able to touch each finger with the thumb of the same hand

ABNORMAL FINDINGS

nerve damage; felon (infection of a fingertip with infection in an adjacent fascial space); tendon sheath infections (tenderness and swelling along the tendon sheath and partial flexion of the affected finger)

Dupuytren's contracture: progressive permanent thickening and contracture of the tendon sheath with resulting fixed flexion of the affected finger and a palpable hard cordlike tendon sheath

Degenerative joint disease: hard painless nodules on the dorsolateral aspects of interphalangeal joints; radial deviation of the distal phalanx; Heberden's nodes on the distal interphalangeal (DIP) joints; Bouchard's nodes on the proximal interphalangeal (PIP) joints; sparing of the metacarpophalangeal (MCP) joints

Gout: asymmetrical involvement of the joints; a knobby swelling that may be hot and painful and may ulcerate and discharge chalky urates; uric acid usually high

Acute rheumatoid arthritis: symmetrical involvement of the joints; tenderness, stiffness; nodules and deformities of the wrist, MCP, and PIP joints with sparing of the DIP joints

Chronic rheumatoid arthritis: chronic swelling and thickening of the MCP and PIP joints; interosseous muscular atrophy of the hand; ulnar deviation of the fingers; nodules, swan neck and boutonnière deformities of the fingers

Hips
Normal ROM:

Flexion with straight knee: 90 degrees

Flexion with knee bent: 110 to 120 degrees

Extension: 30 degrees

Abduction: 45 to 50 degrees

Adduction: 20 to 30 degrees

Internal rotation: 35 to 40 degrees

External rotation: 45 degrees

Arthritis evidenced by pain and limited ROM of the hip

Flexion deformity of the hip: test by flexing the knee on one side and watching for involuntary flexing of the opposite side

Pelvic tilt: unequal height of the ileac crests may be secondary to unequal lengths of the legs or adduction/abduction deformities of the hip

Aseptic necrosis of the hip: secondary to sickle cell disease

Sacroiliac pain: test by having supine patient firmly flex the opposite knee against the abdomen while hyperextending the other extended leg by dangling it off the edge of the examining table

Knees
Normal ROM:

Flexion: 130 degrees

Hyperextension: 15 degrees

Internal rotation: 10 degrees

Bow knees (genu varum), knock knees (genu valgum), Flexion contracture (inability to extend joint fully), bony enlargement (degenerative joint disease)

NORMAL FINDINGS	ABNORMAL FINDINGS
	Tenosynovitis: loss of hollows above and adjacent to patella suggests synovial thickening
	Ballottement of patella suggests synovial thickening or fluid; positive bulge sign (milk upward on the medial side of patella, then tap the lateral side of the patella and watch for returning bulge of fluid)
	Thickening, bogginess, or tenderness suggests synovial inflammation of the knee
	Instability
	Abduction mobility: relaxation or tear of the medial collateral ligament
	Adduction mobility: relaxation or tear of the lateral collateral ligament
	Anterior mobility: anterior cruciate ligament damage
	Posterior mobility: posterior cruciate ligament damage
	Torn medial or lateral meniscus

Ankles
Normal ROM:
    Dorsiflexion: 20 degrees
    Plantar flexion: 45 degrees
    Eversion: 20 degrees
    Inversion: 30 degrees
	Pain, swelling, erythema, or stiffness; arthritis may be difficult to differentiate from edema or cellulitis

Toes
Normal ROM:

Flexion: 35 to 60 degrees (depending on the specific joint)

Extension: 0 to 90 degrees (depending on specific joint)

Abduction: varies

Adduction: normally unable

Rheumatoid nodules; tenderness in the small metatarsophalangeal (MTP) joints is an early sign of rheumatoid arthritis; pain or swelling of the first MTP joint of the great toe suggests gout

Halux valgus: great toe abnormally abducted with medial deviation

Bunion: usually a painful swelling of the MTP joint of the great toe

Flat feet: absence of normal arch of the sole of the foot; the sole lies flat on the floor

Clinical Notes

Be gentle when examining the patient, and take care not to inflict harm by expecting the patient to do more than he or she is capable of. Never force a joint beyond its natural limit while guiding it through passive range of motion or special maneuvers.

In many conditions, the use of imaging modalities such as roentgenography, myelography, or bone scanning may be necessary to confirm suspected diagnosis.

 ## Geriatric Considerations

NORMAL FINDINGS

Muscles — Decline in mass, tone, and strength

Bones and joints — Narrowing of joint spaces due to a thinning of cartilage; bony prominences of the vertebrae and ribs

Iliac crest sharpened as a result of a loss of subcutaneous fat; diminished mobility, flexibility, and range of motion

Clinical Notes

Common arthritic changes of the wrist and knees result in joint enlargement, crepitus, stiffness, and pain.

Shrinking and stiffening of ligaments and tendons and narrowing of joint spaces can limit range of motion. Slowly and gently assess movement of joints to limit pain and potential injury.

 Pediatric Considerations

History

Birth injuries?

History of congenital hip dysplasia in extended family?

Sports?

Trauma?

NORMAL FINDINGS	ABNORMAL FINDINGS
Newborn	
	Postdelivery clavicular fracture
Adduction of the forefoot, may be manipulated to neutral or an overcorrected position	Metatarsus adductus: rigid adduction of forefoot
Equal gluteal folds	
	Congenital hip dysplasia: positive Ortolani sign ("click" heard when hips are flexed and abducted to examining table) and/or limited abduction
Infant	
Bowing of legs, which begins to disappear at 18 months to 2 years	
Fat pad under arch of foot, "flat-footed" appearance	

Child and Adolescent

Wide-based gait with some pronation of feet until age 2 years
Scoliosis: "S" curve of spine; asymmetry of shoulders and hips

Increased lumbar curvature in the toddler, resulting in a protuberant abdomen

Knock-kneed appearance in the preschool child and early school-age child

>3 inches between ankles when knees are together

RAPID ASSESSMENT

THE PATIENT WITH LOW BACK PAIN

How did the pain occur? With exercise? Straining? Lifting? Trauma?

What is the quality of the pain?

Where is the pain located precisely?

Does the pain radiate?

Is the pain reproducible by palpation or by position changes?

Are there associated symptoms of fever, nausea, vomiting, diarrhea, constipation, cough, chest pain, shortness of breath, dysuria, hematuria, oliguria?

Is there associated muscle weakness? What extremities are affected?

Are there parasthesias?

Physical Examination	Rationale
Examine and palpate the back.	Determine whether there is trauma, bruises, lesions, or masses contributing to back pain.
Examine and palpate the spine with patient standing and bending over at the waist.	Determine presence of lesions masses, localized tenderness, abnormal contours of the spine: kyphosis, scoliosis etc.
Examine range of motion and muscle strength of all extremities	Decreased range of motion and muscle strength may indicate herniated disc, compression fracture, mass, infectious process.
Test for sensory deficits in all extremities.	Sensory deficits may indicate lesion, mass, infection, disc disease, compression fracture.
Check for deep tendon reflexes	Reflex defects may indicate disc disease, cord compression, or injury brain tumor, etc.
Check for flank tenderness	May indicate pyelonephritis or renal abscess infection or calculi.
Check urinalysis	Pyuria may indicate urinary tract infection, hematuria may indicate renal or uretheral calculi
Perform pelvic exam	Pelvic infections, abscess, menses, pregnancy often present as low back pain
Rectal and prostate exam	Prostatitis, prostatic hypertrophy, rectal mass, fecal impaction, rectal fissure, fistula, may present as low back pain

Assessment of the Nervous System

HISTORY AND CURRENT STATUS QUESTIONS

Headache?	Location; unilateral or bilateral; character and severity of pain; acute or gradual onset; pattern of occurrence—constant or chronic recurrent, worsening over time or stable in intensity, time of onset, duration, precipitating or associated factors such as particular activities, time of day, or stressful events, effect of movem3ent such as change in head position, coughing or sneezing; associated symptoms such as nausea and vomiting, nasal congestion, fever, relief measures tried and their effectiveness.
Injury?	Description, including any loss of consciousness and its duration; date of occurrence; precipitating or prodromal events such as faintness or pain, treatment; residual effects.
Dizziness/light-headedness?	Frequency; duration; time of occurrence; precipitating factors, such as change in position, or specific activities.
Fainting?	Frequency; duration; time of occurrence; precipitating factors; position at time of occurrence; warning signs; appearance before and after syncope; feeling after return of consciousness.

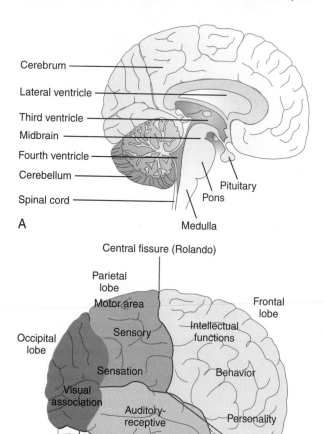

FIGURE 22-1 Anatomy of the central nervous system. *(A)* Main structures of the brain. *(B)* Lobes of the cerebral hemispheres and their specialized functions.

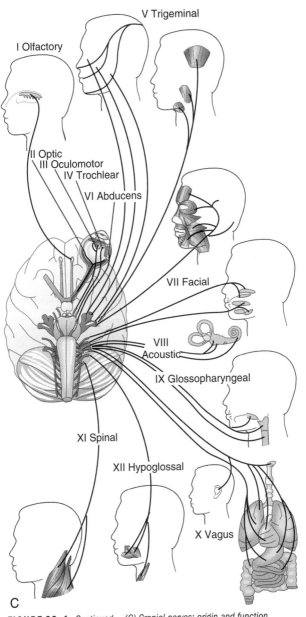

FIGURE 22–1 *Continued.* (C) Cranial nerves: origin and function.

Vertigo (sense you or the room about you is spinning)?	Time and type (sudden or gradual) of onset; severity; constant or intermittent; associated symptoms (nausea, vomiting, ataxia); precipitating factors; type and effectiveness of relief measures used.
Seizures?	Type; sequence of seizure effects on the body, duration; postictal reaction (e.g., sleep, confusion, weakness, headache) and its duration; aura; age at onset; cause if known; frequency, any recent change in frequency; time of last seizure; exacerbating factors (e.g., stress, fatigue, specific activities, omission of medication); treatment; side effects of medication; pattern of compliance with treatment regimen.
Tremors or other involuntary movements?	Date and type of onset; body part(s) affected; exacerbating factors (e.g., purposeful activity, rest, anxiety); ameliorating factors (e.g., rest, activity, alcohol).
Paresis or paralysis?	Date and type of onset; body parts affected; generalized or localized; unilateral or bilateral; type of progression, if any; effect of rest; effect of repeated activity; other exacerbating or ameliorating factors; associated symptoms.
Coordination problems?	Loss of balance when walking; history of falls; clumsy movements; listing to one side; date and type of onset; associated symptoms; exacerbating factors; ameliorating factors.
Paresthesias or loss of sensation	Date and type of onset; type (e.g., tingling, pins and needles); area of body affected; constant or intermittent; effect on daily activities; exacerbating factors; ameliorating factors.
Difficulty speaking?	Type (e.g., difficulty forming words, saying what is meant); date and type of onset; constant or intermittent; exacerbating factors; ameliorating factors; associated symptoms.

Difficulty swallowing?	Solids and/or liquids; drooling; type and time of onset; constant or intermittent; exacerbating factors; ameliorating factors; associated symptoms.
History of nervous system disease?	Type of disorder (e.g., stroke, spinal cord injury, meningitis, encephalitis); date of occurrence; treatment; residual effects.
Medications? (OTC and prescription)	Name; dose; route; frequency; reason for use.
Use of alcohol?	Type; amount (glasses, bottles, pint, half pint); frequency (e.g., daily, two to three times per week, two to three times per month); pattern of use (weekends only, when out or with company, with dinner, evenings, morning); type and frequency of any "hangover" symptoms; occurrence of blackout periods.
Drug abuse?	Type of drug(s) used; route; amount; frequency; length of time used; effects; date and type of any treatment.
Exposure to environmental or occupational hazards?	Type of hazard; type and duration of exposure.

PHYSICAL EXAMINATION

Equipment

Cotton; flashlight; newspaper (or other printed material); ophthalmoscope; otoscope; reflex hammer; sterile needle; Snellen chart; tape measure; tongue depressor; tuning fork; various objects of different shapes (key, marble, coin); vials (stoppered) containing peppermint, coffee, or other familiar aromatic substances, salt or vinegar, and hot and cold water.

Procedures, Techniques, and Findings

Assess mental status

See Chapter 5.

Assess speech and language function

Expressive component of speech

Ask patient to repeat one or two phrases. Note clarity, fluency and ability to repeat the phrases without hesitancy or substitution.

Show the patient five different objects and ask him or her to name each.

Receptive component of speech

Ask the patient to follow a simple one-step command such as "Close your eyes."

Assess cranial nerve (Table 22–1) function

CN I (olfactory nerve)

TABLE 22–1	Functions of the Cranial Nerves	
Cranial Nerve	**Sensory Function**	**Motor Function**
I Olfactory	Smell	
II Optic	Sight	
III Oculomotor		Extraocular eye movements, elevation of lids, pupillary constriction, control of lens shape
IV Trochlear		Downward and inward eye movement
V Trigeminal	Sensation of face, scalp, oral and nasal mucous membranes and the cornea	Chewing movements of the jaw
VI Abducens		Lateral eye movement
VII Facial	Taste on the anterior 2/3 of the tongue	Facial movement, eye closure, labial speech
VIII Acoustic	Hearing and balance	
IX Glosso-pharyngeal	Taste on the posterior third of the tongue, pharyngeal gag reflex, sensation from the ear drum and ear canal	Swallowing and phonation muscles of the pharynx
X Vagus	Sensation from pharynx, viscera, carotid body, carotid sinus	Swallowing and talking muscles of the palate, pharynx, larynyx
XI Spinal		Trapezius and sternocleido-mastoid muscle movement
XII Hypoglossal		Tongue movement

Ask the patient to close his or her eyes.

Occlude one of the patient's nostrils.

Hold a familiar aromatic substance such as coffee, vanilla, peppermint, or tobacco under the nonoccluded nostril.

Ask the patient to sniff and identify the odor.

Repeat for the other nostril.

Note unilateral or bilateral decrease or loss of smell.

Repeat with a different familiar aromatic substance to determine if the patient can distinguish a difference between odors.

Test only when patient complains of loss of smell or when assessing for an intracranial lesion.

CN II (optic nerve)

Test visual acuity and visual fields (see Chapter 7).

Examine the retina with an ophthalmoscope (see Chapter 7).

CN III, IV, and VI (oculomotor, trochlear, and abducens nerves)

Check pupils for size, regularity, equality, reaction to light, and accommodation.

Test extraocular movements by having the patient follow your finger as you move it through the six cardinal positions of gaze. Note limited or abnormal movement (see Chapter 7).

CN V (trigeminal nerve)

Motor function

Ask the patient to clench the teeth.

Palpate the temporal and masseter muscles (Fig. 22–2) and push down on the chin to try and separate the jaws while the teeth are clenched (see Fig. 7–3).

Note decreased strength or asymmetric jaw movement.

Sensory function

Check light touch sensation in all three sensory divisions of the trigeminal nerve: ophthalmic, maxillary, mandibular (Fig. 22–3)

Ask the patient to close his or her eyes.

Proceed to alternately touch a cotton wisp or sterile pin to the patient's right forehead, cheek, and chin.

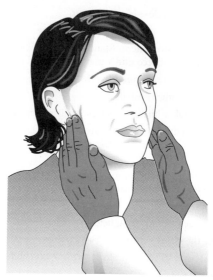

FIGURE 22-2 Palpation of the masseter muscles to check motor function of CN V (trigeminal nerve).

Ask patient to identify what is felt and where.

Repeat for the left side.

Note absent, decreased, or unequal sensation.

Check the corneal reflex (also tests motor function of CN VII)

Ask patient to remove contact lenses, if worn.

Direct patient to look straight ahead.

Bring a wisp of cotton in from the side and lightly touch the cornea (not just the conjunctiva) of each eye in turn (Fig. 22–4).

Observe for bilateral blinking.

Omit in a routine screening examination.

CN VII (facial nerve)

Sensory function

Test taste

Touch the anterior tongue on both sides with a cotton applicator that has been dipped in a sugar, salt, or lemon solution.

Ask the patient to identify the taste.

Omit in a routine screening examination.

Motor function

Ask the patient to smile, frown, raise the eyebrows, show upper and lower teeth, keep eyes tightly closed as you try to open them (see Fig. 7–2), and puff out the cheeks.

Observe for mobility and symmetry as these actions are performed.

Press puffed cheeks in and note if air escapes equally from both sides.

CN VIII (acoustic nerve)

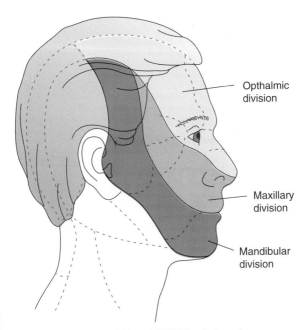

Opthalmic division

Maxillary division

Mandibular division

FIGURE 22-3 Sensory divisions of CN V (trigeminal nerve).

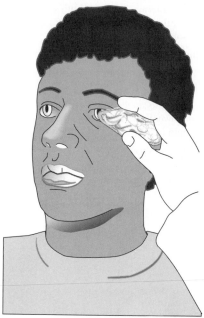

FIGURE 22-4 Checking the corneal reflex.

Test hearing (see Chapter 9).

CN IX and X (glossopharyngeal and vagus nerves)

Ask patient to open the mouth and say "ah" as you depress the tongue with a tongue blade.

Note movement of the uvula, soft palate, and tonsillar pillars.

Touch the tongue blade to the posterior pharyngeal wall.

Observe for gagging.

Note quality of patient's voice.

CN XI (spinal accessory nerve)

Inspect the right and left sternocleidomastoid and trapezius muscles for equal size.

Place your hand against the side of the patient's chin and face (Fig. 22–5A).

Ask patient to turn head against this resistance.

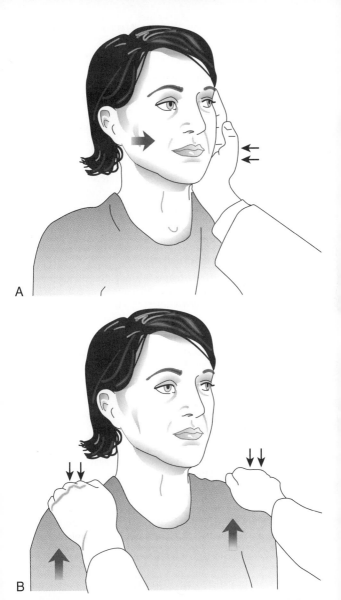

FIGURE 22-5 Checking function of CN XI (spinal accessory nerve) *(A)* by asking the patient to turn the head against the resistance of the examiner's hand placed on the side of the face and chin; *(B)* by having the patient shrug shoulders against the resistance of the examiner's hands.

Repeat for the opposite side.

Place your hands on the patient's shoulders.

Direct patient to shrug shoulders against the resistance of your hands (Fig. 22–5B).

Compare movement on right and left sides for equality.

CN XII (hypoglossal nerve)

Direct the patient to stick out the tongue.

Observe direction of protrusion and note any movement or wasting.

Ask patient to say "late date night."

Assess motor function (see Chapter 21)

Muscle mass and size

Ask patient to lie down and relax.

Inspect and palpate each muscle group, comparing muscles on the right side of the body with counterparts on the left side. Verify any perceived differences in size with a tape measure.

Muscle tone

Passively move each extremity through a full range of motion, noting any hypotonia or hypertonia (see Chapter 21).

Movement

Check voluntary and involuntary movement and range of motion (see Chapter 21).

Muscle strength

Ask patient to move each muscle group against your resistance (see Chapter 21).

Compare left side to right side and note symmetry and equality of strength.

Grade motor strength against gravity and resistance on a scale of 0 to 5, with 5 being normal and 0 complete paralysis (Table 22–2).

Gait

Observe the patient walk 10 to 20 feet away from you, turn, and return.

TABLE 22-2	Grading Scale for Motor Strength
Grade	**Description**
5/5	Normal muscle strength (i.e., full range of motion against examiner resistance)
4/5	Full range of motion of muscle that can be overcome with increased examiner resistance
3/5	Full range of motion of muscle against gravity only; is overcome with slight examiner resistance
2/5	Weak movement of muscle but insufficient to overcome gravity
1/5	Slight visible or palpable contraction muscle noted but no movement results
0/5	Complete paralysis

Note posture, rhythm, effort, symmetry of gait, and coordination of arm movement and arm swing.

Ask patient to walk heel to toe (tandem walk) along a straight line (Figure 22–6).

Assess balance and coordination

Romberg's test

Have patient stand with feet together and arms at sides.

Direct patient to close eyes and maintain the position.

Wait 20 seconds and then tell the patient to open the eyes and relax.

Be prepared to catch the patient during this test if he or she should start to fall.

Arm drift test (Pronator drift)

Ask patient to put both arms straight out in front of the body with palms up, close the eyes, and hold this arm position for 10 to 15 seconds. Watch for any downward drift of the arms or pronation of the hands (Fig. 22–7).

Rapid alternating movement (RAM) test

Ask the patient to touch the right thumb to each finger of the right hand, going from index finger to little finger and back to the index finger.

Have patient repeat the action using the left hand.

OR

Ask patient to place the palms of the hands on the knees; lift the hands; turn them over; and touch the knees with the back of the hands.

Direct the patient to repeat this action as rapidly as possible (Fig. 22–8).

Finger-to-finger test

Ask the patient to touch your index finger and then his or her own nose with his or her right and then left index finger (Fig. 22–9).

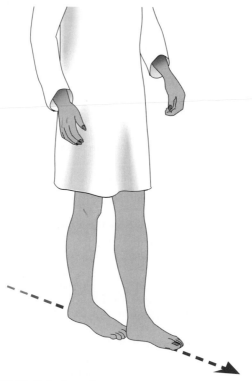

FIGURE 22-6 Tandem walk.

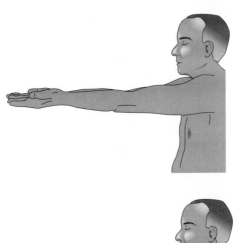
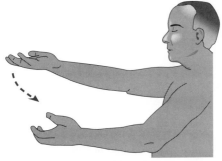

FIGURE 22-7 Arm drift (pronator drift) test.

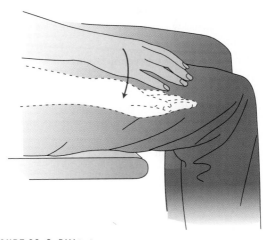

FIGURE 22-8 RAM test.

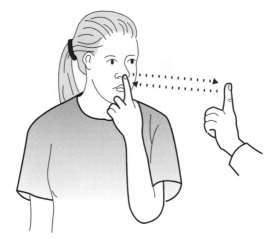

FIGURE 22-9 Finger-to-finger test.

Finger-to-nose test

Ask patient to extend arms in front of him- or herself, close his or her eyes and touch the tip of the nose with the right and then the left index finger (Fig. 22–10).

Direct the patient to continue to perform this alternating motion as quickly as possible.

Heel-to-shin test

Have the patient assume a dorsal recumbent position.

Direct the patient to place the heel of the right foot just below the knee on the left shin and run the heel down the shin to the ankle (Fig. 22–11).

Have the patient repeat the procedure with the left heel on the right shin.

Assess sensory function

Light touch

Ask patient to close eyes then stroke an area of the patient's skin with a wisp of cotton.

Ask the patient to identify the area touched and to describe the feeling.

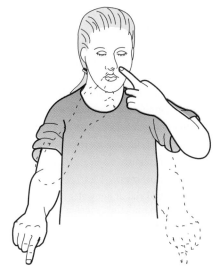

FIGURE 22-10 Finger-to-nose test.

Repeat on the opposite side of the body and compare results.

Repeat this procedure in a systematic manner, testing the hands, forearms, upper arms, torso, thigh, lower leg, and foot.

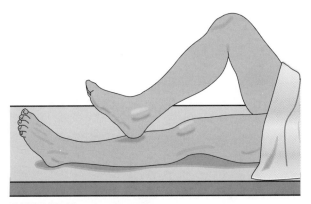

FIGURE 22-11 Heel-to-shin test.

Superficial pain sensation

Ask patient to close eyes.

Gently touch the point of a sterile needle against the skin.

Randomly intersperse touches with the blunt end of the needle.

Allow at least 2 seconds between each touch.

Ask patient to indicate if sharpness or dullness is felt.

Progress in a systematic fashion as for light touch.

Dispose of used needle in a sharps container.

Temperature sensitivity

Ask patient to close eyes.

Touch a stoppered vial of hot water to the patient's abdomen for 1 second, then touch a vial of cold water to the abdomen for 1 second.

Ask the patient to state which was hot and cold.

Repeat for the extremities.

Position sense

Ask patient to close eyes.

Move the fingers and toes up or down, one by one.

Ask the patient to state in which direction the digit has been moved (Fig. 22–12).

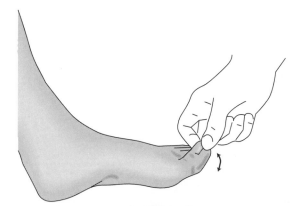

FIGURE 22-12 Testing position sense.

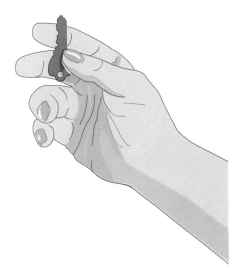

FIGURE 22-13 Stereognosis.

Check three or four digits on each hand and foot.

Vibration sense

Ask patient to close eyes.

Tap the tines of a tuning fork on the heel of your hand to set it vibrating.

Place it firmly over the distal interphalangeal joint of the patient's finger.

Ask the patient what he or she feels.

Repeat for the distal joint of the patient's great toe.

Test more proximal bony prominences if vibration sense is impaired.

Stereognosis

Ask the patient to close his or her eyes.

Place a familiar object, such as a key, in the patient's hands (Fig. 22–13).

Ask the patient to name it.

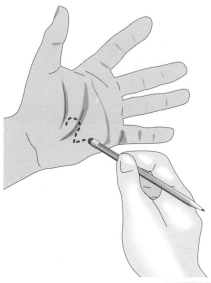

FIGURE 22-14 Graphesthesia.

Repeat for the other hand using a different familiar object, such as a coin.

Graphesthesia

Ask the patient to close his or her eyes.

Trace a single number or letter on the palm of the patient's hand with a blunt object, such as the cap of a pen (Fig. 22–14).

Ask the patient to identify what was traced.

Repeat for the other hand using different numbers or letters.

Two-point discrimination

Touch two sterile needles to two places on the skin simultaneously.

Repeat the touch, moving the needles more and more closely together until the patient no longer feels separate points.

Record the last distance between the needles.

Extinction

Touch the same area on the right and left side of the body simultaneously.

Ask patient where and how many touches were felt.

Point location

Touch skin quickly.

Ask the patient to put the finger where the skin was just touched.

Assess reflexes

Deep tendon reflexes (DTRs)

Use a reflex hammer (Fig. 22–15A, B, C) to strike the muscle's insertion tendon and thus stimulate the reflex.

Make certain the limb is relaxed but the muscle is slightly stretched.

Biceps reflex

Facing the patient, place the forearm to be tested over the forearm of your nondominant hand.

Place the thumb of your nondominant hand over the biceps tendon and support the patient's elbow with the rest of your hand.

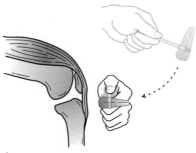

A

FIGURE 22-15 *(A)* Reflex hammer with motion indicated and the muscle that it is going to impact. *Illustration continued on following page*

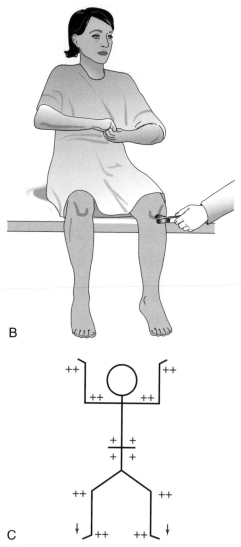

B

C

FIGURE 22-15 *Continued. (B)* Reinforcement. *(C)* Stick drawing showing documentation of reflex activity.

Strike your thumb with the pointed end of the reflex hammer (Fig. 22–16).

Observe for flexion of the forearm.

Repeat on other arm.

Triceps reflex

Hold the patient's arm across the chest with the elbow bent by grasping the wrist or hold the inner aspect of the patient's upper arm just above the antecubital space so the elbow is bent and the forearm and hand hang down.

Tell the patient to let the arm go "dead."

Strike the triceps tendon with the pointed end of the reflex hammer just above the elbow (Fig. 22–17).

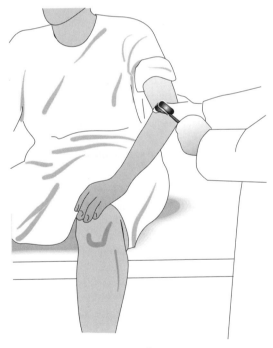

FIGURE 22-16 Testing the biceps reflex.

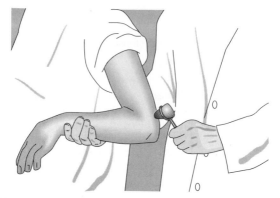

FIGURE 22-17 Testing the triceps reflex.

Observe for extension of the forearm.

Repeat on patient's other arm.

Brachioradialis reflex

Have the patient rest the hands with the ulnar side down, thumb side up, in the lap.

Strike the forearm 2 to 3 cm above the radial styloid process with the pointed end of the reflex hammer (Fig. 22–18).

Observe for flexion and supination of the forearm.

Repeat on other arm.

Patellar (knee-jerk) reflex

Ask the patient to sit and dangle the legs freely over the side of the examining table or bed.

Place your nondominant hand across the patient's leg just above the knee.

Strike the tendon just below the patella with the wide end of the reflex hammer (Fig. 22–19).

Observe for extension of the lower leg and feel for contraction of the quadriceps.

If the patient is unable to sit up and dangle the legs, flex the patient's knee by placing your nondominant arm under it.

Support the weight by bracing your hand on top of the patient's other leg just above the knee.

Achilles reflex

Flex the patient's knee and externally rotate the hip, and dorsiflex the foot.

Strike the Achilles tendon with the wide end of the reflex hammer (Fig. 22–20).

Feel for plantar flexion of the foot in your hand.

Test for clonus especially if reflexes are hyperactive

Place one hand under the calf to support the lower leg.

Dorsiflex the foot briskly with the other hand and hold it in dorsiflexion.

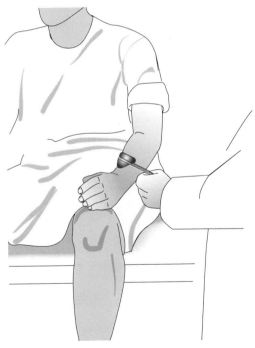

FIGURE 22-18 Testing the brachioradialis reflex.

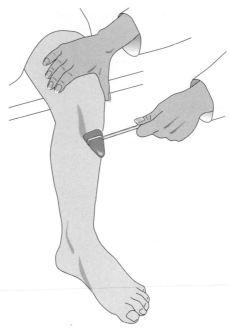

FIGURE 22-19 Testing the patellar reflex.

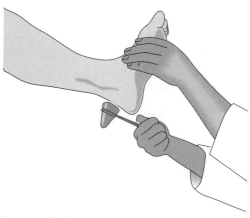

FIGURE 22-20 Testing the achilles reflex.

Observe and feel for rapid rhythmic contractions of the foot.

Superficial reflexes (receptors in skin)

Ask the patient to lie flat on the back with the knees slightly bent.

Upper and lower abdominal

Stroke the skin with the handle of the reflex hammer, moving from the side of the abdomen into the midline. Do this on the right and left side of the upper (below the rib cage and above the umbilicus) and lower (above the symphysis pubis) abdomen (Fig. 22–21A).

Observe for contraction of the abdominal muscle on the side stroked accompanied by deviation of the umbilicus to that same side.

If the patient is obese, pull the skin to the opposite side and feel for it to pull back toward the side stroked.

Cremasteric reflex

Use the handle of the reflex hammer to stroke the inner aspect of the male thigh (Fig. 22–21B).

Observe for elevation of the testicle on the side stroked.

Plantar reflex

Use the handle of the reflex hammer to stroke the lateral side of the sole of the foot and across the ball of the foot, forming an upside down "J" (Fig. 22–22).

Observe for plantar flexion of toes or foot.

NORMAL FINDINGS	ABNORMAL FINDINGS
Mental status speech and language	
See Chapter 5	See Chapter 5
Expressive speech function	
Follows simple directions	Unable to follow simple directions
Responds to complex commands without demonstration	Unable to respond to complex demands without demonstration

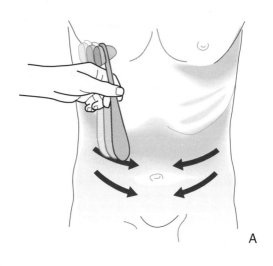

A

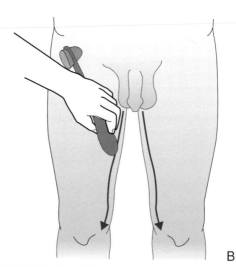

B

FIGURE 22-21 Testing; *(A)* Abdominal reflexes. *(B)* Cremasteric reflex.

NORMAL FINDINGS	**ABNORMAL FINDINGS**

Receptive speech function

Repeats phrases clearly, fluently

Hesitates, uses substitute words, speech unclear

Identifies common objects correctly by name

Cannot identify common objects, or identifies by function, not name

Cranial nerve function
CN I (olfactory nerve)

Common odors are correctly identified using each side of the nose

Decreased or loss of smell (anosmia) unilaterally or bilaterally

CN II (optic nerve)

Visual field intact

Visual field loss
Papilledema, optic atrophy

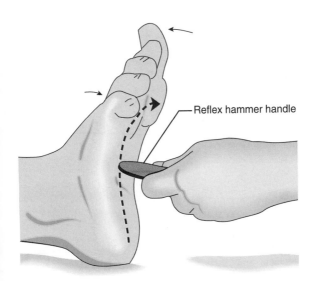

FIGURE 22-22 Plantar reflex.

NORMAL FINDINGS	ABNORMAL FINDINGS

CN III, IV, VI (oculomotor, trochlear, and abducens nerves)

PERRLA	Ptosis, pupillary abnormalities (Table 22–2), deviated gaze, limited eye movement, nystagmus (other than end point)

CN V (trigeminal nerve)

Motor function

Symmetric jaw movement	Asymmetric jaw movement
Equal muscle strength on left and right sides sufficient to prevent examiner from separating jaw	Unilateral or bilateral decreased strength

Sensory function

Sensations of light touch, dullness, and sharpness perceived over forehead, cheeks, and chin	Absent, decreased, or unequal sensation
Eyelids blink when cornea touched with cotton (also reflects motor function of CN VII)	Absent blink

CN VII (facial nerve)

Motor function

Symmetrical strength and movement of facial muscles	Loss of or asymmetric movement
	Muscle weakness suggested by loss of nasolabial fold, droopy side of face, or drooping of lower lid, no escape of air from one or both cheeks

Sensory function

Correctly identifies salt, sweet, sour, and bitter taste	Unable to identify salty, sweet, sour, and/or bitter taste

CN VIII (acoustic nerve)

Hearing acuity within normal range	Unilateral or bilateral hearing impairment (see Chapter 9)

CN IX and X (glossopharyngeal and vagus nerves)

Motor function

Uvula and soft palate rise in midline and tonsillar pillars move medially when patient says "ah"	Absence or asymmetry of movement Deviated uvula
Voice smooth	Voice hoarse or strained
Gag reflex intact	Absence of gag reflex

CN XI (spinal accessory nerve)

Muscle strength equal on left and right	Muscle weakness or paralysis

CN XII (hypoglossal nerve)

Tongue is midline when protruded, lingual sounds clear, nonpurposeful movement is absent	Wasting, tremors tongue deviates to side Indistinct, lingual speech sounds

Motor function

Muscle mass and size

Symmetrical size (muscles on dominant side may be somewhat larger than those on the nondominant side)	Unilateral or bilateral atrophy or marked hypertrophy

Muscle tone

Mild, even resistance to movement	Flacidity, decreased resistance, spasticity, rigidity

Movement

Equal on both sides, normal range of motion	Limited movement bilaterally or unilaterally

Muscle strength

Approximately equal on both sides	Marked asymmetric strength

NORMAL FINDINGS	ABNORMAL FINDINGS
Balance and coordination	
Gait	
Smooth, rhythmic, effortless swing of arms coordinated with step of opposite legs, able to walk a straight line	Stiffness, staggering, reeling, lack of arm swing, unequal rhythm of steps, abnormally wide base of support, scraping of toe or slapping of foot on floor
	Inability to walk a straight line
Romberg's test	
Position maintained with no more than slight swaying	Swaying, falling, weakening of base of support
Rapid alternating movements	
Rapid, smooth, accurate movement	Slow, clumsy, jerky, uncoordinated movement
Arm drift	
No drift	Downward drift or pronation
Finger-to-finger test	
Smooth, accurate movement	Misses the nose or finger
Finger-to-nose test	
Smooth, accurate movement	Misses nose, jerky movements
Heel-to-shin test	
Smoothly moves heel in a straight line down the shin	Heel falls off shin
Sensory function	
Light touch	
Touch sensation intact	Increased, decreased or absent touch sensation
Superficial pain sensation	
Sensations are correctly identified as sharp or dull	Sensations are not perceived or are incorrectly identified as sharp or dull

Temperature sensitivity

Hot and cold temperatures are correctly identified	Inability to distinguish hot from cold

Position sense

Direction of digit movement is correctly identified	Digit movement not detected

Vibration sense

Vibration perceived equally	Vibration not perceived

Stereognosis

Object is correctly named	Object is not correctly named

Graphesthesia

Number is correctly identified	Number is not correctly identified

Two-point discrimination

2 to 8 mm in fingertips 40 to 75 mm on upper arms, thighs, and back	Increase in minimal distance at which two points are perceived

Extinction

Sensations felt on both sides of the body	Absent or unilateral sensation

Point location

Area of skin touched can be identified	Area of skin touched unable to be identified

Deep tendon reflexes

Biceps reflex

Flexion of the forearm	Hypo- or hyperreflexia

Triceps reflex

Extension of the forearm	Hypo- or hyperreflexia

Brachioradialis reflex

Flexion and supination of the forearm	Hypo- or hyperreflexia

Quadriceps reflex

Extension of the lower leg	Hypo- or hyperreflexia

Achilles reflex

Plantar flexion of the foot	Hypo- or hyperreflexia

NORMAL FINDINGS	ABNORMAL FINDINGS

Clonus

No movement	Rapid rhythmic contractions of the foot

Superficial reflexes

Upper and lower abdominal reflex

Ipsilateral contraction of the abdominal muscle accompanied by deviation of the umbilicus toward the stimulated side	Absence of muscular contraction

Cremasteric reflex

Ipsilateral elevation of the testicle	Absence of testicular elevation

Plantar reflex

Plantar flexion of the toes or foot	Dorsiflexion of the great toe and fanning of all toes (positive Babinski sign)

Clinical Note

To determine changes in neurologic baseline quickly assess as follows:

Level of consciousness	Assess orientation to person, place, time, and reality.
	Assess appropriateness of speech; note clarity and fluency.
Cranial nerves	Assess pupillary response to light bilaterally (oculomotor nerve).
	Assess extraocular movements: oculomotor, trochlear, and abducens nerves.
	Assess facial symmetry (facial nerve).
	Assess gag reflex (glossopharyngeal nerve).
	Assess tongue in midline when extended (hypoglossal nerve).
Motor function	Assess arm drifting.
	Assess handgrip.
	Assess straight-leg raise.
	Assess knee bends.

	Assess ankle plantar flexion and dorsiflexion.
Sensory function	Assess sensation to light touch and pinprick in extremities and on trunk, comparing right with left sides.

Geriatric Considerations

NORMAL FINDINGS

Reflexes	Reaction time and response to stimuli slowed. Gag, ankle, abdominal and plantar reflexes may be diminished or absent.

Also see geriatric considerations in Chapters 5, 8, 9, and 21.

Clinical Note

Changes of the nervous system attributable to aging are generally symmetrical. If asymmetric, investigate for cause other than aging.

Pediatric Considerations

History

Pregnancy and birth history?

Quality of cry?

Developmental history: meeting age-appropriate milestones?

Abnormal sucking or eye movements?

"Absence" spells?

Accident, injuries, ingestions?

Family history of metabolic, genetic, or any progressive neurologic condition? Seizure disorders?

Physical Examination

Observe for newborn reflexes, then age-appropriate suppression

Note infant's level of alertness and arousability

Note infant's position/posturing

Test vision and hearing in the age-appropriate manner

Equipment

Bell

Findings

NORMAL FINDINGS	ABNORMAL FINDINGS
Newborn	

Crying but consolable	
Intermittent fussiness	Extreme irritability, not consolable
	High-pitched "cat's cry"
Newborn reflexes present:	
Disappears at approximately:	Newborn reflexes asymmetric, absent, or persisting beyond expected time of disappearance
Crawling 1–2 mos	
Dance 1–2 mos	
Tonic neck 4–6 mos	
Moro 4–6 mos	
Grasp (palmer and plantar) 3–4 mos	
+ Babinski 1–2 yrs	
Rooting and sucking 3–4 mos	
Neck righting 10 mos	
Symmetric muscle tone, bulk, and movement; rapid recoil after extension	
Fine tremors of short duration	Asymmetry
Ankle clonus	Flaccidity
	Tremors that cannot be quieted by the examiner
	Stiffness
	Extension
	Spastic adduction
	Athetosis
Fontanelles soft and flat	
Various sizes	Bulging or markedly depressed

Hearing:

| May respond by opening eyes wide, blinking, ceasing or initiating movement, or turning to sound | No response |

Infant

   Reflexes

      Neck righting (4–6 mos)

      Parachute (8–9 mos)

   Separation anxiety when removed from primary caretaker (9 mos)

Child

   Cerebral dominance (3–4 yrs)

| *Clear speech (90% understandable other than by primary care-taker)* | Unclear speech |

RAPID ASSESSMENT

THE PATIENT WITH DIZZINESS

Ask the patient to describe the dizziness

Is the patient lightheaded, near fainting?

Does the patient feel the room spinning around him or feel pulled in one direction?

Does the patient have tinnitus (ringing in the ears)?

Was there any preceeding trauma?

Are there associated symptoms of fever, headache, nausea, vomiting, diarrhea?

Are there palpitations or chest pain?

Is the patient short of breath?

Does the patient have a productive cough?

Are vital signs stable: blood pressure, pulse, respirations, temperature?

When does the dizziness occur?

How is it relieved?

Is there any syncope, associated seizure activity, or change in mental status?

Is the patient anemic or actively bleeding?

Has the patient lost weight, been dieting?

Is the patient undergoing an emotional crisis? Having a conversion reaction?

Is there associated muscle weakness?

Is the patient pregnant?

Does the patient have any underlying systemic disease?

Has the patient been taking any new medications, drugs, alcohol?

Has the patient recently changed any routine medication dosages?

Physical Examination	Rationale
Check vital signs	Hypotension, bradycardia, bradypnea, tachypnea, and fever may all cause dizziness
Check pulse oximetry	Hypoxia may cause dizziness
Check electrolytes and routine labs	Hypoglycemia, dehydration, anemia, infections
Examine the head and palpate the skull for trauma, lesions, abnormalities	Head trauma, lacerations, may cause dizziness

Continued on next page

Physical Examination	Rationale
Examine the eyes and vision	Fundoscopic exam may reveal signs of hypertension, diabetes, glaucoma. Vision changes may cause dizziness.
Examine the ear and hearing	Check for tinnitus, infection, impaction, foreign body. Check for hearing deficit.
Examine the nose and sinuses	Upper respiratory infectiton and sinusitis may cause dizziness
Examine the pharynx	Check for tonsillitis, strep throat, epiglottitis, peritonsilar abscess, dental decay
Examine the neck	Check for lymphadenopathy indicating infection or mass, JVD—congestive heart failure, thyroid tenderness, mass or enlargement, tracheal deviation (pneumothorax or effusion)
Examine the chest and lungs	Check for absent or abnormal breath sounds indicating pneumothorax, effusions, pneumonia, pleurisy, bronchitis. All contribute to hypoxia which can cause dizziness.
Examine the heart	Abnormal rate and rhythm may indicate a serious arrythmia and inadequate cardiac output which can cause dizziness
Examine the abdomen	Check for distention, tenderness, obstruction, rebound tenderness, pulsatile mass, bruits, GI bleed, pyelonephritis, abscess hepatitis, pancreatitis, UTI, cystitis, bleeding ulcer
Perform neuro examination including cranial nerves, muscle tone, strength, sensation, and gait	

Recommended Immunization Schedules for Children and Adults in the United States

Recommended Childhood Immunization Schedule United States, January–December 2001

Vaccines[1] are listed under routinely recommended ages. Bars indicate range of recommended ages for immunization. Any dose not given at the recommended age should be given as a "catch-up" immunization at any subsequent visit when indicated and feasible. Ovals indicate vaccines to be given if previously recommended doses were missed or given earlier than the recommended minimum age.

Age ▶ Vaccines ▼	Birth	1 mo	2 mos	4 mos	6 mos	12 mos	15 mos	18 mos	24 mos	4-6 yrs	11-12 yrs	14-16 yrs
Hepatitis B[2]		Hep B #1	Hep B #2			Hep B # 3					Hep B[2]	
Diphtheria, Tetanus, Pertussis[3]			DTaP	DTaP	DTaP		DTaP[3]			DTaP	Td	
H. influenzae type b[4]			Hib	Hib	Hib	Hib						
Inactivated Polio[5]			IPV	IPV		IPV[5]				IPV[5]		
Pneumococcal Conjugate[6]			PCV	PCV	PCV	PCV						
Measles, Mumps, Rubella[7]						MMR				MMR[7]	MMR[7]	
Varicella[8]						Var					Var[8]	
Hepatitis A[9]									Hep A—in selected areas[9]			

Approved by the Advisory Committee on Immunization Practices (ACIP), the American Academy of Pediatrics (AAP), and the American Academy of Family Physicians (AAFP).

From www.medem.com/MedLB/

For additional information on vaccines and their use, go to the website.

428

Summary of Adolescent/Adult Immunization Recommendations

AGENT

Tetanus, Diptheria Toxoids Combined (Td)	Influenza Vaccine	Pneumococcal Polysaccharide Vaccine (PPV)
INDICATIONS		
All adults	a. Adults 50 years of age and older.	a. Adults 65 years of age and older.
All adolescents should be assessed at 11-12 or 14-16 years of age and immunized if no dose was received during the previous 5 years.	b. Residents of nursing homes or other facilities for patients with chronic medical conditions.	b. Persons ≥2 years with chronic cardiovascular or pulmonary disorders including congestive heart failure, diabetes mellitus, chronic liver disease, alcoholism, CSF leaks, cardiomyopathy, COPD or emphysema.
	c. Persons ≥6 mo of age with chronic cardiovascular or pulmonary disorders, including asthma.	c. Persons ≥2 years with splenic dysfunction or asplenia, hematologic malignancy, multiple myeloma, renal failure, organ transplantation or immunosuppressive conditions, including HIV infection.
	d. Persons ≥6 mo of age with chronic metabolic diseases (including diabetes), renal dysfunction, hemoglobinopathies, immunosuppressive or immunodeficiency disorders.	d. Alaskan Natives and certain American Indian populations.
	e. Women in their 2nd or 3rd trimester of pregnancy during influenza season.	
	f. Persons 6 months–18 years of age receiving long-term aspirin therapy.	
	g. Groups, including household members and care givers, who can infect high risk persons.	

Table continued on following page

Summary of Adolescent/Adult Immunization Recommendations *Continued*

AGENT		
Tetanus, Diptheria Toxoids Combined (Td)	Influenza Vaccine	Pneumococcal Polysaccharide Vaccine (PPV)
PRIMARY SCHEDULE Two doses 4-8 weeks apart, third dose 6-12 months after the second. No need to repeat doses if the schedule is interrupted. **Dose:** 0.5 mL intramuscular (IM) **Booster:** At 10-year intervals throughout life.	**Dose:** 0.5 mL intramuscular (IM) Given annually, each fall.	One dose for most people* **Dose:** 0.5 mL intramuscular (IM) or subcutaneous (SC) *Persons vaccinated prior to age 65 should be vaccinated at age 65 if 5 or more years have passed since the first dose. For all persons with functional or anatomic asplenia, transplant patients, patients with chronic kidney disease, immunosuppressed or immunodeficient persons, and others at highest risk of fatal infection, a second dose should be given—at least 5 years after first dose.

Measles and Mumps Vaccines**	Rubella Vaccine**	Hepatitis B Vaccine
INDICATIONS		
a. Adults born after 1956 without written documentation of immunization on or after the first birthday.	a. Persons (especially women) without written documentation of immunization on or after the first birthday or of seropositivity.	a. Persons with occupational risk of exposure to blood or blood-contaminated body fluids.
b. Health care personnel born after 1956 who are at risk of exposure to patients with measles should have documentation of two doses of vaccine on or after the first birthday or of measles seropositivity.	b. Health care personnel who are at risk of exposure to patients with rubella and who may have contact with pregnant patients should have at least one dose.	b. Clients and staff of institutions for the developmentally disabled.
		c. Hemodialysis patients.
c. HIV-infected persons without severe immunosuppression.		d. Recipients of clotting-factor concentrates.
		e. Household contacts and sex partners of those chronically infected with HBV.
d. Travelers to foreign countries.		f. **Family members of adoptees from countries where HBV infection is endemic, if adoptees are HBsAg+.**
e. Persons entering post-secondary educational institutions (e.g., college).		g. Certain international travelers.
		h. Injecting drug users.
		i. Men who have sex with men.
		j. Heterosexual men and women with multiple sex partners or recent episode of a sexually transmitted disease.
		k. Inmates of long-term correctional facilities.
		l. All unvaccinated adolescents.

**These vaccines can be given in the combined form measles-mumps-rubella (MMR). Persons already immune to one or more components can still receive MMR.

Table continued on following page

Summary of Adolescent/Adult Immunization Recommendations *Continued*

AGENT

Measles and Mumps Vaccines**	Rubella Vaccine**	Hepatitis B Vaccine
PRIMARY SCHEDULE	One dose.	Three doses: second dose 1-2 months after the first, third dose 4-6 months after the first.
At least one dose. (Two doses of **measles-containing vaccine** if in college, in health care profession or traveling to a foreign country with second dose at least 1 month after the first.)	**Dose:** 0.5 mL subcutaneous (SC)	No need to start series over if schedule interrupted. Can start series with one manufacturer's vaccine and finish with another.
Dose: 0.5 mL subcutaneous (SC)		**Dose (Adult):** intramuscular (IM) Recombivax HB®: 10 :g/1.0 mL (green cap) Engerix-B®: 20 :g/1.0 mL (orange cap)
		Dose (Adolescents 11-19 years): intramuscular (IM) Recombivax HB®: 5 :g/0.5 mL (yellow cap) Engerix-B®: 10 :g/0.5 mL (light blue cap) **Booster:** None presently recommended.

*These vaccines can be given in the combined form measles-mumps-rubella (MMR). Persons already immune to one or more components can still receive MMR.

Poliovirus Vaccine: IPV–Inactivated OPV–Oral (Live)	Varicella Vaccine	Hepatitis A Vaccine
INDICATIONS		
Routine vaccination of those ≥18 years of age residing in the U.S. is not necessary. Vaccination is recommended for the following high-risk adults:	a. Persons of any age without a reliable history of varicella disease or vaccination, or who are seronegative for varicella.	a. Persons traveling to or working in countries with high or intermediate endemicity of infection
a. Travelers to areas or countries where poliomyelitis is epidemic or endemic.	b. **Susceptible adolescents and adults living in households with children.**	b. Men who have sex with men.
b. Members of communities or specific population groups with disease caused by wild polioviruses.	c. All susceptible health care workers.	c. Injecting and non-injecting illegal drug users.
c. Laboratory workers who handle specimens that may contain polioviruses.	d. Susceptible family contacts of immunocompromised persons.	d. Persons who work with HAV-infected primates or with HAV in a research laboratory setting.
d. Health care workers who have close contact with patients who may be excreting wild polioviruses.	e. Susceptible persons in the following groups who are at high risk for exposure: –persons who live or work in environments in which transmission of varicella is likely (e.g., teachers of young children, day care employees, residents and staff in institutional settings) or can occur (e.g., college students, inmates and staff of correctional institutions, military personnel)	e. Persons with chronic liver disease.
e. Unvaccinated adults whose children will be receiving OPV.	–nonpregnant women of childbearing age –international travelers	f. Persons with clotting factor disorders. g. Consider food handlers, where determined to be cost-effective by health authorities or employers.

Table continued on following page

433

Summary of Adolescent/Adult Immunization Recommendations *Continued*

AGENT

Poliovirus Vaccine: IPV–Inactivated OPV–Oral (Live)	Varicella Vaccine	Hepatitis A Vaccine
PRIMARY SCHEDULE		
Unimmunized adolescents/adults:	For persons <13 years of age, one dose.	HAVRIX®: Two doses, separated by 6-12 months.
IPV is recommended—two doses at 4-8 week intervals, third dose 6-12 months after second (can be as soon as 2 months).	For persons 13 years of age and older, two doses separated by 4-8 weeks. If >8 weeks elapse following the first dose, the second dose can be administered without restarting the schedule.	Adults (19 years of age and older) **Dose:** 1.0 mL intramuscular (IM)
Dose: 0.5 mL subcutaneous (SC) or intramuscular (IM).	**Dose:** 0.5 mL subcutaneous (SC)	Persons 2-18 years of age **Dose:** 0.5 mL (IM).
Partially immunized adolescents/adults: Complete primary series with IPV (IPV schedule shown above).		VAQTA®: Adults (18 years of age and older): Two doses, separated by 6 months **Dose:** 1.0 mL intramuscular (IM)
OPV is *no longer recommended for use in the United States.*		Persons 2-17 years of age: Two doses, separated by 6-18 months **Dose:** 0.5 mL (IM)

Adapted from the recommendations of the Advisory Committee on Immunization Practices (ACIP). Foreign travel and less commonly used vaccines such as typhoid, rabies, and meningococcal are not included.

For additional information in these immunizations go to www.CDC.gov.

Standard Precautions

Use Standard Precautions, or the equivalent, for the care of all patients. *Category IB*

A. Handwashing
1. Wash hands after touching blood, body fluids, secretions, excretions, and contaminated items, whether or not gloves are worn. Wash hands immediately after gloves are removed, between patient contacts, and when otherwise indicated to avoid transfer of microorganisms to other patients or environments. It may be necessary to wash hands between tasks and procedures on the same patient to prevent cross-contamination of different body sites. *Category IB*
2. Use a plain (nonantimicrobial) soap for routine hand-washing. *Category IB*
3. Use an antimicrobial agent or a waterless antiseptic agent for specific circumstances (e.g., control of outbreaks or hyperendemic infections), as defined by the infection control program. *Category IB* (See Contact Precautions for additional recommendations on using antimicrobial and antiseptic agents.)

B. Gloves
Wear gloves (clean, nonsterile gloves are adequate) when touching blood, body fluids, secretions, excretions, and contaminated items. Put on clean gloves just before touching mucous membranes and nonintact skin. Change gloves between tasks and procedures on the same patient after contact with material that may contain a high concentration of microorganisms. Remove gloves promptly after use, before

touching noncontaminated items and environmental surfaces, and before going to another patient, and wash hands immediately to avoid transfer of microorganisms to other patients or environments. *Category IB*

C. Mask, Eye Protection, Face Shield

Wear a mask and eye protection or a face shield to protect mucous membranes of the eyes, nose, and mouth during procedures and patient-care activities that are likely to generate splashes or sprays of blood, body fluids, secretions, and excretions. *Category IB*

D. Gown

Wear a gown (a clean, nonsterile gown is adequate) to protect skin and to prevent soiling of clothing during procedures and patient-care activities that are likely to generate splashes or sprays of blood, body fluids, secretions, or excretions. Select a gown that is appropriate for the activity and amount of fluid likely to be encountered. Remove a soiled gown as promptly as possible, and wash hands to avoid transfer of microorganisms to other patients or environments. *Category IB*

E. Patient-Care Equipment

Handle used patient-care equipment soiled with blood, body fluids, secretions, and excretions in a manner that prevents skin and mucous membrane exposures, contamination of clothing, and transfer of microorganisms to other patients and environments. Ensure that reusable equipment is not used for the care of another patient until it has been cleaned and reprocessed appropriately. Ensure that single-use items are discarded properly. *Category IB*

F. Environmental Control

Ensure that the hospital has adequate procedures for the routine care, cleaning, and disinfection of environmental surfaces, beds, bedrails, bedside equipment, and other frequently touched surfaces, and ensure that these procedures are being followed. *Category IB*

G. Linen

Handle, transport, and process used linen soiled with blood, body fluids, secretions, and excretions in a manner that prevents skin and mucous membrane exposures and contamination of clothing, and that avoids transfer of microorganisms to other patients and environments. *Category IB*

H. Occupational Health and Bloodborne Pathogens

1. Take care to prevent injuries when using needles, scalpels, and other sharp instruments or devices; when handling

sharp instruments after procedures; when cleaning used instruments; and when disposing of used needles. Never recap used needles, or otherwise manipulate them using both hands, or use any other technique that involves directing the point of a needle toward any part of the body; rather, use either a one-handed "scoop" technique or a mechanical device designed for holding the needle sheath. Do not remove used needles from disposable syringes by hand, and do not bend, break, or otherwise manipulate used needles by hand. Place used disposable syringes and needles, scalpel blades, and other sharp items in appropriate puncture-resistant containers, which are located as close as practical to the area in which the items were used, and place reusable syringes and needles in a puncture-resistant container for transport to the reprocessing area. *Category IB*

2. Use mouthpieces, resuscitation bags, or other ventilation devices as an alternative to mouth-to-mouth resuscitation methods in areas where the need for resuscitation is predictable. *Category IB*

I. Patient Placement
Place a patient who contaminates the environment or who does not (or cannot be expected to) assist in maintaining appropriate hygiene or environmental control in a private room. If a private room is not available, consult with infection control professionals regarding patient placement or other alternatives. *Category IB*

For further information on precautions, go to http://www.cdc.gov/ncidod/hip/isolat/isopart2.htm

From the Public Health Service, US Department of Health and Human Services, Centers for Disease Control and Prevention, Atlanta, Georgia.
Garner JS, Hospital Infection Control Practices Advisory Committee. Guideline for isolation precautions in hospitals. Infect Control Hosp Epidemiol 1996;17:53–80, and Am J Infect Control 1996;24:24–52.

Signs of Abuse

Consider the possibility of physical abuse when a patient presents with:

a history of repeated accidents or trauma.

concealed or unexplained injuries.

an apparent discrepancy between the history of trauma and the type of injury incurred.

acute embarrassment over a seemingly non-embarrassing incident.

 GERIATRIC CONSIDERATIONS

Consider the possibility of abuse of the elderly when the patient presents with:

signs of physical trauma such as fingerprint bruises on the upper arms, bruises on the inner thighs, or other unexplained injuries.

signs of neglect such as dirty, long nails; matted hair; thick corns and calluses; soiled clothing; body or mouth odor.

signs of psychological abuse such as reports of long periods of isolation.

PEDIATRIC CONSIDERATIONS

Abuse is suspected and/or diagnosed by identifying a combination of signs and symptoms. The only *single* symptom that validates sexual abuse is confirmed STD in an otherwise sexually inactive child. Possible signs of physical abuse in a child include:

Failure to thrive

Unexplained injuries

Injuries where the explanation does not fit the type of injury

Bruises in various stages of healing especially in areas other than those where children frequently bang themselves when playing

Multiple fractures

Cigarette burns

Burns on lower extremities, hands, and buttocks

Behavior and emotional problems

Poor school performance

Decreased attention span

Aggravated fears

Possible signs of sexual abuse in a child include:

Precocious sexual knowledge and/or play

Genital, throat, and/or anal STD's

Trauma to the genitalia

Behavior and emotional problems

Poor school performance

Aggravated fears

Decreased attention span

Clinical Note

Obtain an uncoached history from a child or adolescent in his/her own words.

From Monahan, F.D. et al. Nursing Care of Adults. Philadelphia; WB Saunders, 1994.

Height and Weight Tables

Height and Weight Table for Women

Height Feet Inches	Small Frame	Medium Frame	Large Frame
4'10"	102-111	109-121	118-131
4'11"	103-113	111-123	120-134
5'0"	104-115	113-126	122-137
5'1"	106-118	115-129	125-140
5'2"	108-121	118-132	128-143
5'3"	111-124	121-135	131-147
5'4"	114-127	124-138	134-151
5'5"	117-130	127-141	137-155
5'6"	120-133	130-144	140-159
5'7"	123-136	133-147	143-163
5'8"	126-139	136-150	146-167
5'9"	129-142	139-153	149-170
5'10"	132-145	142-156	152-173
5'11"	135-148	145-159	155-176
6'0"	138-151	148-162	158-179

Weights at ages 25–59 based on lowest mortality. Weight in pounds according to frame (in indoor clothing weighing 3 lbs.; shoes with 1" heels).

Height and Weight Table for Men

Height Feet Inches	Small Frame	Medium Frame	Large Frame
5'2"	128-134	131-141	138-150
5'3"	130-136	133-143	140-153
5'4"	132-138	135-145	142-156
5'5"	134-140	137-148	144-160
5'6"	136-142	139-151	146-164
5'7"	138-145	142-154	149-168
5'8"	140-148	145-157	152-172
5'9"	142-151	148-160	155-176
5'10"	144-154	151-163	158-180
5'11"	146-157	154-166	161-184
6'0"	149-160	157-170	164-188
6'1"	152-164	160-174	168-192
6'2"	155-168	164-178	172-197
6'3"	158-172	167-182	176-202
6'4"	162-176	171-187	181-207

Weights at ages 25–59 based on lowest mortality. Weight in pounds according to frame (in indoor clothing weighing 5 lbs.; shoes with 1" heels).

Height and Weight Measurements for Girls

	Height by Percentiles						Weight by Percentiles					
	5		50		95		5		50		95	
Age*	cm	inches	cm	inches	cm	inches	kg	lb	kg	lb	kg	lb
Birth	45.4	17¾	49.9	19¾	52.9	20¾	2.36	5¼	3.23	7	3.81	8½
3 months	55.4	21¾	59.5	23½	63.4	25	4.18	9¼	5.4	12	6.74	14¾
6 months	61.8	24¼	65.9	26	70.2	27¾	5.79	12¾	7.21	16	8.73	19¼
9 months	66.1	26	70.4	27¾	75.0	29½	7.0	15½	8.56	18¾	10.17	22½
1	69.8	27½	74.3	29¼	79.1	31¼	7.84	17¼	9.53	21	11.24	24¾
1½	76.0	30	80.9	31¾	86.1	34	8.92	19¾	10.82	23¾	12.76	28¼
2†	81.6	32¼	86.8	34¼	93.6	36¾	9.95	22	11.8	26	14.15	31¼
2½†	84.6	33¼	90.0	35½	96.6	38	10.8	23¾	13.03	28¾	15.76	34¾
3	88.3	34¾	94.1	37	100.6	39½	11.61	25½	14.1	31	17.22	38
3½	91.7	36	97.9	38½	104.5	41¼	12.37	27¼	15.07	33¼	18.59	41

4	95.0	37½	101.6	40	108.3	42¾	13.11	29	15.96	35¼	19.91	44
4½	98.1	38½	105.0	41¼	112.0	44	13.83	30½	16.81	37	21.24	46¾
5	101.1	39¾	108.4	42¾	115.6	45½	14.55	32	17.66	39	22.62	49¾
6	106.6	42	114.6	45	122.7	48¼	16.05	35½	19.52	43	25.75	56¾
7	111.8	44	120.6	47½	129.5	51	17.71	39	21.84	48¼	29.68	65½
8	116.9	46	126.4	49¾	136.2	53½	19.62	43¼	24.84	54¾	34.71	76½
9	122.1	48	132.2	52	142.9	56¼	21.82	48	28.46	62¾	40.64	89½
10	127.5	50¼	138.3	54½	149.5	58¾	24.36	53¾	32.55	71¾	47.17	104
11	133.5	52½	144.8	57	156.2	61½	27.24	60	36.95	81½	54.0	119
12	139.8	55	151.5	59¾	162.7	64	30.52	67¼	41.53	91½	60.81	134
13	145.2	57¼	157.1	61¾	168.1	66¼	34.14	75¼	46.1	101¾	67.3	148¼
14	148.7	58½	160.4	63¼	171.3	67½	37.76	83¼	50.28	110¾	73.08	161
15	150.5	59¼	161.8	63¾	172.8	68	40.99	90¼	53.68	118¼	77.78	171½
16	151.6	59¾	162.4	64	173.3	68¼	43.41	95¾	55.89	123¼	80.99	178½
17	152.7	60	163.1	64¼	173.5	68¼	44.74	98¾	56.69	125	82.46	181¾
18	153.6	60½	163.7	64½	173.6	68¼	45.26	99¾	56.62	124¾	82.47	181¾

Modified from National Center for Health Statistics (NCHS), Health Resources Administration. Department of Health, Education and Welfare, Hyattsville, MD. Conversion of metric data to approximate inches and pounds by Ross Laboratories.

**Years unless otherwise indicated.*

†Height data include some recumbent length measurements, which make values slightly higher than if all measurements had been of stature.

From Whaley & Wong. Nursing Care of Infants and Children, 6e. Mosby, 1999.

Height and Weight Measurements for Boys

	Height by Percentiles						Weight by Percentiles					
	5		50		95		5		50		95	
Age*	cm	inches	cm	inches	cm	inches	kg	lb	kg	lb	kg	lb
Birth	46.4	18¼	50.5	20	54.4	21½	2.54	5½	3.27	7¼	4.15	9¼
3 months	56.7	22¼	61.1	24	65.4	25¾	4.43	9¾	5.98	13¼	7.37	16¼
6 months	63.4	25	67.8	26¾	72.3	28½	6.20	13¾	7.85	17¼	9.46	20¼
9 months	68.0	26¾	72.3	28½	77.1	30¼	7.52	16½	9.18	20¼	10.93	24
1	71.7	28¼	76.1	30	81.2	32	8.43	18½	10.15	22½	11.99	26½
1½	77.5	30½	82.4	32½	88.1	34¾	9.59	21¼	11.47	25¼	13.44	29½
2†	82.5	32½	86.8	34¼	94.4	37¼	10.49	23¼	12.34	27¼	15.50	34¼
2½†	85.4	33½	90.4	35½	97.8	38½	11.27	24¾	13.52	29¾	16.61	36½
3	89.0	35	94.9	37¼	102.0	40¼	12.05	26½	14.62	32¼	17.77	39¼
3½	92.5	36½	99.1	39	106.1	41¾	12.84	28¼	15.68	34½	18.98	41¼

4	95.8	37¾	102.9	40½	109.9	43¼	13.64	30	16.69	36¾	20.27	44¼
4½	98.9	39	106.6	42	113.5	44¾	14.45	31¾	17.69	39	21.63	47¼
5	102.0	40¼	109.9	43¼	117.0	46	15.27	33¾	18.67	41¼	23.09	51
6	107.7	42½	116.1	45¾	123.5	48½	16.93	37¼	20.69	45½	26.34	58
7	113.0	44½	121.7	48	129.7	51	18.64	41	22.85	50¼	30.12	66½
8	118.1	46½	127.0	50	135.7	53½	20.40	45	25.30	55¾	34.51	76
9	122.9	48½	132.2	52	141.8	55¾	22.25	49	28.13	62	39.58	87¼
10	127.7	50¼	137.5	54¼	148.1	58¼	24.33	53¾	31.44	69¼	45.27	99¼
11	132.6	52¼	143.3	56½	154.9	61	26.80	59	35.30	77¾	51.47	113½
12	137.6	54¼	149.7	59	162.3	64	29.85	65¾	39.78	87¾	58.09	128
13	142.9	56¼	156.5	61½	169.8	66¾	33.64	74¼	44.95	99	65.02	143¼
14	148.8	58½	163.1	64¼	176.7	69½	38.22	84¼	50.77	112	72.13	159
15	155.2	61	169.0	66½	181.9	71½	43.11	95	56.71	125	79.12	174½
16	161.1	63½	173.5	68¼	185.4	73	47.74	105¼	62.10	137	85.62	188¼
17	164.9	65	176.2	69¼	187.3	73¾	51.50	113½	66.31	146¼	91.31	201¼
18	165.7	65¼	176.8	69½	187.6	73¾	53.97	119	68.88	151¾	95.76	211

Modified from National Center for Health Statistics (NCHS), Health Resources Administration. Department of Health, Education and Welfare, Hyattsville, MD. Conversion of metric data to approximate inches and pounds by Ross Laboratories.

Author's note: As of this writing, the Centers for Disease Control and Prevention, National Center for Health Statistics (NCHS), has published revised growth charts for the United States. The 14 NCHS growth charts and new body mass index-for-age (BMI-for-age) charts are available for boys and girls from birth to age 20 years. The growth charts can be printed from the website: www.cdc.gov/growthcharts.

**Years unless otherwise indicated.*

†Height data include some recumbent length measurements, which make values slightly higher than if all measurements had been of stature (standing height).

From Whaley & Wong. Nursing Care of Infants and Children, 6e. Mosby, 1999.

Daily Requirements of Basic Food Groups

	Women and Some Older Adults	Children, Teen Girls, Active Women, Most Men	Teen Boys and Active Men
Calorie level*	about 1,600	about 2,200	about 2,800
Bread group	6	9	11
Vegetable group	3	4	5
Fruit group	2	3	4
Milk group	**2–3	**2–3	**2–3
Meat group	2, for a total of 5 ounces	2, for a total of 6 ounces	3, for a total of 7 ounces

*These are the calorie levels if you choose lowfat, lean foods from the 5 major food groups and use foods from the fats, oils, and sweets group sparingly.

**Women who are pregnant or breastfeeding, teenagers, and young adults to age 24 need 3 servings.

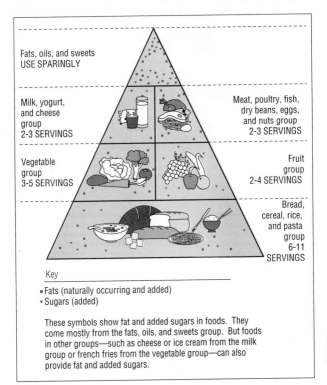

Key
- Fats (naturally occurring and added)
- Sugars (added)

These symbols show fat and added sugars in foods. They come mostly from the fats, oils, and sweets group. But foods in other groups—such as cheese or ice cream from the milk group or french fries from the vegetable group—can also provide fat and added sugars.

The Food Guide Pyramid
A Guide to Daily Food Choices

Normal Laboratory Values

Reference Intervals in Hematology

	Conventional Units	SI Units
Acid hemolysis test (Ham)	No hemolysis	No hemolysis
Alkaline phosphatase, leukocyte	Total score 14-100	Total score 14-100
Cell counts		
Erythrocytes		
Males	4.6-6.2 million/mm^3	4.6-6.2 × 10^{12}/L
Females	4.2-5.4 million/mm^3	4.2-5.4 × 10^{12}/L
Children (varies with age)	4.5-5.1 million/mm^3	4.5-5.1 × 10^{12}/L
Leukocytes, total	4500-11,000 mm^3	4.5-11.0 × 10^9/L
Leukocytes, differential counts		Absolute
		0/L
Myelocytes	0%	0/L
Band neutrophils	3-5%	150-400 × 10^6/L
Segmented neutrophils	54-62%	3000-5800 × 10^6/L
Lymphocytes	25-33%	1500-3000 × 10^6/L
Monocytes	3-7%	300-500 × 10^6/L
Eosinophils	1-3%	50-250 × 10^6/L
Basophils	0%	15-50 × 10^6/L
Platelets	150,000-400,000/mm^3	150-400 × 10^9/L

Table continued on following page

Reference Intervals in Hematology *Continued*

	Conventional Units	SI Units
Reticulocytes	25,000–75,000/mm³ (0.5–1.5% of erythrocytes)	25–75 × 10⁹/L
Coagulation tests		
Bleeding time (template)	2.75–8.0 min	2.75–8.0 min
Coagulation time (glass tube)	5–15 min	5–15 min
D dimer	<0.5 µg/mL	<0.5 mg/L
Factor VIII and other coagulation factors	50–150% of normal	0.5–1.5 of normal
Fibrin split products (Thrombo-Welco test)	<10 µg/mL	<10 mg/L
Fibrinogen	200–400 mg/dL	2.0–4.0 gm/L
Partial thromboplastin time activated (aPTT)	20–35 s	20–35 s
Prothrombin time (PT)	12.0–14.0 s	12.0–14.0 s
Coombs' test		
Direct	Negative	Negative
Indirect	Negative	Negative
Corpuscular values of erythrocytes		
Mean corpuscular hemoglobin (MCH)	26–34 pg/cell	26–34 pg/cell
Mean corpuscular volume (MCV)	80–96 µm³	80–96 fL
Mean corpuscular hemoglobin concentration (MCHC)	32–36 gm/dL	320–360 gm/L
Haptoglobin	20–165 mg/dL	0.20–1.65 gm/L

Hematocrit		
Males	40-54 mL/dL	0.40-0.54
Females	37-47 mL/dL	0.37-0.47
Newborns	49-54 mL/dL	0.49-0.54
Children (varies with age)	35-49 mL/dL	0.35-0.49
Hemoglobin		
Males	13.0-18.0 gm/dL	8.1-11.2 mmol/L
Females	12.0-16.0 gm/dL	7.4-9.9 mmol/L
Newborns	16.5-19.5 gm/dL	10.2-12.1 mmol/L
Children (varies with age)	11.2-16.5 gm/dL	7.0-10.2 mmol/L
Hemoglobin, fetal	<1.0% of total	<0.01 of total
Hemoglobin A_{1c}	3-5% of total	0.03-0.05 of total
Hemoglobin A_2	1.5-3.0% of total	0.015-0.03 of total
Hemoglobin, plasma	0-5.0 mg/dL	0.0-3.2 μmol/L
Methemoglobin	30-130 mg/dL	19-80 μmol/L
Sedimentation rate (ESR)		
Wintrobe: Males	0-5 mm/h	0-5 mm/h
Females	0-15 mm/h	0-15 mm/h
Westergren: Males	0-15 mm/h	0-15 mm/h
Females	0-20 mm/h	0-20 mm/h

Reference Intervals* for Clinical Chemistry (Blood, Serum, and Plasma)

	Conventional Units	SI Units
Acetoacetate plus acetone		
Qualitative	Negative	Negative
Quantitative	0.3–2.0 mg/dL	30–200 nmol/L
Acid phosphatase, serum (thymolphthalein monophosphate)	0.1–0.6 U/L	0.1–0.6 U/L
ACTH (see Corticotropin)		
Alanine aminotransferase (ALT), serum (SGPT)	1–45 U/L	1–45 U/L
Albumin, serum	3.3–5.2 gm/dL	33–52 gm/L
Aldolase, serum	0.0–7.0 U/L	0.0–7.0 U/L
Aldosterone, plasma		
Standing	5–30 ng/dL	140–830 pmol/L
Recumbent	3–10 ng/dL	80–275 pmol/L
Alkaline phosphatase (ALP), serum		
Adult	35–150 U/L	35–150 U/L
Adolescent	100–500 U/L	100–500 U/L
Child	100–350 U/L	100–350 U/L
Ammonia nitrogen, plasma	10–50 μmol/L	10–50 μmol/L
Amylase, serum	25–125 U/L	25–125 U/L
Anion gap, serum, calculated	8–16 mEq/L	8–16 mmol/L
Ascorbic acid, blood	0.4–1.5 mg/dL	23–85 μmol/L
Aspartate aminotransferase (AST), serum (SGOT)	1–36 U/L	1–36 U/L

Base excess, arterial blood, calculated	0 ± 2 mEq/L	0 ± 2 mmol/L
Bicarbonate		
Venous plasma	23–29 mEq/L	23–29 mmol/L
Arterial blood	21–27 mEq/L	21–27 mmol/L
Bile acids, serum	0.3–3.0 mg/dL	0.8–7.6 μmol/L
Bilirubin, serum		
Conjugated	0.1–0.4 mg/dL	1.7–6.8 μmol/L
Total	0.3–1.1 mg/dL	5.1–19 μmol/L
Calcium, serum	8.4–10.6 mg/dL	2.25–2.75 mmol/L
Calcium, ionized, serum	4.25–5.25 mg/dL	2.10–2.65 mmol/L
Carbon dioxide, total, serum or plasma	24–31 mEq/L	24–31 mmol/L
Carbon dioxide tension (P_{CO_2}), blood	35–45 mmHg	35–45 mmHg
β-Carotene, serum	60–260 μg/dL	1.1–8.6 μmol/L
Ceruloplasmin, serum	23–44 mg/dL	230–440 mg/L
Chloride, serum or plasma	96–106 mEq/L	96–106 mmol/L
Cholesterol, serum or EDTA plasma		
Desirable range	<200 mg/dL	<5.20 mmol/L
LDL cholesterol	60–180 mg/dL	1.55–4.65 mmol/L
HDL cholesterol	30–80 mg/dL	0.80–2.05 mmol/L
Copper	70–140 μg/dL	11–22 μmol/L
Corticotropin (ACTH), plasma, 8 A.M.	10–80 pg/mL	2–18 pmol/L

*For some procedures, the reference values may vary depending on the method used.

Table continued on following page

453

Reference Intervals* for Clinical Chemistry (Blood, Serum, and Plasma) Continued

	Conventional Units	SI Units
Cortisol, plasma		
8 A.M.	6–23 µg/dL	170–635 nmol/L
4 P.M.	3–15 µg/dL	80–410 nmol/L
10 P.M.	<50% of 8 A.M. value	<0.5 of 8 A.M. value
Creatine, serum		
Males	0.2–0.5 mg/dL	15–40 µmol/L
Females	0.3–0.9 mg/dL	25–70 µmol/L
Creatine kinase (CK), serum		
Males	55–170 U/L	55–170 U/L
Females	30–135 U/L	30–135 U/L
Creatine kinase MB isozyme, serum	<5% of total CK activity	<5% of total CK activity
	<5% ng/mL by immuno-assay	<5% ng/mL by immuno-assay
Creatinine, serum	0.6–1.2 mg/dL	50–110 µmol/L
Estradiol-17β, adult		
Males	10–65 pg/mL	35–240 pmol/L
Females		
Follicular	30–100 pg/mL	110–370 pmol/L
Ovulatory	200–400 pg/mL	730–1470 pmol/L
Luteal	50–140 pg/mL	180–510 pmol/L
Ferritin, serum	20–200 ng/mL	20–200 µg/L

Fibrinogen, plasma	200–400 mg/dL	2.0–4.0 g/L
Folate, serum	3–18 ng/mL	6.8–41 nmol/L
Erythrocytes	145–540 ng/mL	330–1220 nmol/L
Follicle-stimulating hormone (FSH), plasma		
Males	4–25 mU/mL	4–25 U/L
Females, premenopausal	4–30 mU/mL	4–30 U/L
Females, postmenopausal	40–250 mU/mL	40–250 U/L
Gamma-Glutamyltransferase (GTT), serum	5–40 U/L	5–40 U/L
Gastrin, fasting serum	0–100 pg/mL	0–100 ng/L
Glucose, fasting, plasma or serum	70–115 mg/dL	3.9–6.4 mmol/L
Growth hormone (hGH), plasma, adult, fasting	0–6 ng/mL	0–6 µg/L
Haptoglobin, serum	20–165 mg/dL	0.20–1.65 g/L
Iron, serum	75–175 µg/dL	13–31 µmol/L
Iron binding capacity, serum		
Total	250–410 µg/dL	45–73 µmol/L
Saturation	20–55%	0.20–0.55
Lactate		
Venous whole blood	5.0–20.0 mg/dL	0.6–2.2 mmol/L
Arterial whole blood	5.0–15.0 mg/dL	0.6–1.7 mmol/L
Lactate dehydrogenase (LD), serum	100–190 U/L	100–190 U/L

Table continued on following page

Reference Intervals* for Clinical Chemistry (Blood, Serum, and Plasma) Continued

	Conventional Units	SI Units
Lipase, serum	10–140 U/L	10–140 U/L
Lutropin (LH), serum		
Males	1–9 U/L	1–9 U/L
Females		
Follicular phase	2–10 IU/L	2–10 U/L
Mid-cycle peak	15–65 U/L	15–65 U/L
Luteal phase	1–12 U/L	1–12 U/L
Postmenopausal	12–65 U/L	12–65 U/L
Magnesium, serum	1.3–2.1 mg/dL	0.65–1.05 mmol/L
Osmolality	275–295 mOsm/kg water	275–295 mmol/kg water
Oxygen, blood, arterial, room air		
Partial pressure (Pa_{O_2})	80–100 mmHg	80–100 mmHg
Saturation (Sa_{O_2})	95–98%	95–98%
pH, arterial blood	7.35–7.45	7.35–7.45
Phosphate, inorganic, serum		
Adult	3.0–4.5 mg/dL	1.0–1.5 mmol/L
Child	4.0–7.0 mg/dL	1.3–2.3 mmol/L

	Conventional	SI
Potassium		
Serum	3.5–5.0 mEq/L	3.5–5.0 mmol/L
Plasma	3.5–4.5 mEq/L	3.5–4.5 mmol/L
Progesterone, serum, adult		
Males	0.0–0.4 ng/mL	0.0–1.3 μg/L
Females		
Follicular phase	0.1–1.5 ng/mL	0.3–4.8 mmol/L
Luteal phase	2.5–28.0 ng/mL	8.0–89.0 mmol/L
Prolactin, serum		
Males	1.0–15.0 ng/mL	1.0–15.0 μg/L
Females	1.0–20.0 ng/mL	1.0–20.0 μg/L
Protein, serum, electrophoresis		
Total	6.0–8.0 gm/dL	60–80 gm/L
Albumin	3.5–5.5 gm/dL	35–55 gm/L
Globulins		
Alpha$_1$	0.2–0.4 gm/dL	2–4 gm/L
Alpha$_2$	0.5–0.9 gm/dL	5–9 gm/L
Beta	0.6–1.1 gm/dL	6–11 gm/L
Gamma	0.7–1.7 gm/dL	7–17 gm/L
Pyruvate, blood	0.3–0.9 mg/dL	0.03–0.10 mmol/L
Rheumatoid factor	0.0–30.0 IU m/L	0.0–30.0 KIU/L
Sodium, serum or plasma	136–145 mEq/L	136–145 mmol/L

Table continued on following page

Reference Intervals* for Clinical Chemistry (Blood, Serum, and Plasma) *Continued*

	Conventional Units	SI Units
Testosterone, plasma		
Males, adult	275–875 ng/dL	9.5–30 nmol/L
Females, adult	23–75 ng/dL	0.8–2.6 nmol/L
Pregnant females	38–190 ng/dL	1.3–6.6 nmol/L
Thyroglobulin	3–42 ng/mL	3–42 µg/L
Thyrotropin (hTSH), serum	0.4–4.8 µIU/mL	0.4–4.8 mIU/L
Thyrotropin-releasing hormone (TRH)	5–60 pg/mL	5–60 ng/L
Thyroxine (FT$_4$), free, serum	0.9–2.1 ng/dL	12–27 pmol/L
Thyroxine (T$_4$), serum	4.5–12.0 µg/dL	58–154 nmol/L
Triglycerides, serum, after 12-hour fast	40–150 mg/dL	0.4–1.5 g/L
Triiodothyronine (T$_3$), serum	70–190 ng/dL	1.1–2.9 nmol/L
Triiodothyronine uptake, resin (T$_3$RU)	25–38%	0.25–0.38
Urate, serum		
Males	2.5–8.0 mg/dL	150–480 µmol/L
Females	2.2–7.0 mg/dL	130–420 µmol/L
Urea, serum or plasma	24–49 mg/dL	4.0–8.2 mmol/L
Urea nitrogen, serum or plasma	11–23 mg/dL	8.0–16.4 mmol/L
Viscosity, serum	1.4–1.8 × water	1.4–1.8 × water
Vitamin A, serum	20–80 µg/dL	0.70–2.80 µmol/L
Vitamin B$_{12}$, serum	180–900 pg/mL	133–664 pmol/L

Reference Intervals* for Clinical Chemistry (Urine)

	Conventional Units	SI Units
Acetone and acetoacetate, qualitative	Negative	Negative
Albumin		
Qualitative	Negative	Negative
Quantitative	10–100 mg/24 h	0.15–1.5 μmol/day
Aldosterone	3–20 μg/24 h	8.3–55 nmol/day
δ-Aminolevulinic acid	1.3–7.0 mg/24 h	10–53 μmol/day
Amylase	<17 U/h	<17 U/h
Amylase/creatinine clearance ratio	0.01–0.04	0.01–0.04
Bilirubin, qualitative	Negative	Negative
Calcium (regular diet)	<250 mg/24 h	<6.3 nmol/day
Catecholamines		
Epinephrine	<10 μg/24 h	<55 nmol/day
Norepinephrine	<100 μg/24 h	<590 nmol/day
Total free catecholamines	4–126 μg/24 h	24–745 nmol/day
Total metanephrines	0.1–1.6 mg/24 h	0.5–8.1 μmol/day
Chloride (varies with intake)	110–250 mEq/24 h	110–250 mmol/day
Copper	0–50 μg/24 h	0.0–0.80 μmol/day

For some procedures, the reference values may vary depending on the method used.

Table continued on following page

459

Reference Intervals* for Clinical Chemistry (Urine) _Continued_

	Conventional Units	SI Units
Cortisol, free	10–100 µg/24 h	27.6–276 nmol/24 h
Creatinine	15–25 mg/kg	0.13–0.22 mmol/kg/day
Creatine		
Males	0–40 mg/24 h	0.0–0.30 mmol/day
Females	0–80 mg/24 h	0.0–0.60 mmol/day
Creatinine clearance (endogenous)		
Males	110–150 mL/min/1.73 m^2	110–150 ml/min/1.73 m^2
Females	105–132 mL/min/1.73 m^2	105–132 ml/min/1.73 m^2
Dehydroepiandrosterone		
Males	0.2–2.0 mg/24 h	0.7–6.9 µmol/day
Females	0.2–1.8 mg/24 h	0.7–6.2 µmol/day
Estrogens, total		
Males	4–25 µg/24 h	14–90 nmol/day
Females	5–100 µg/24 h	18–360 nmol/day
Glucose (as reducing substance)	<250 mg/24 h	<250 mg/day
Hemoglobin and myoglobin, qualitative	Negative	Negative
Homogentisic acid, qualitative	Negative	Negative
17-Ketogenic steroids		
Males	5–23 mg/24 h	17–80 µmol/day
Females	3–15 mg/24 h	10–52 µmol/day

17-Hydroxycorticosteroids		
Males	3–9 mg/24 h	8.3–25 μmol/day
Females	2–8 mg/24 h	5.5–22 μmol/day
5-Hydroxyindoleacetic acid		
Qualitative	Negative	Negative
Quantitative	2–6 mg/24 h	10–31 μmol/day
17-Ketosteroids		
Males	8–22 mg/24 h	28–76 μmol/day
Females	6–15 mg/24 h	21–52 μmol/day
Magnesium	6.0–10 mEq/24 h	3–5 mmol/day
Metanephrines	0.05–1.2 ng/mg creatine	0.05–1.2 ng/mg creatine
Osmolality	38–1400 mOsm/kg water	38–1400 mOsm/kg water
pH	4.6–8.0	4.6–8.0
Phenylpyruvic acid, qualitative	Negative	Negative
Phosphate	0.4–1.3 grams/24 h	13–42 mmol/day
Porphobilinogen		
Qualitative	Negative	Negative
Quantitative	<2 mg/24 h	<9 μmol/day
Porphyrins		
Coproporphyrin	50–250 μg/24 h	77–380 nmol/day
Uroporphyrin	10–30 μg/24 h	12–36 nmol/day
Potassium	25–125 mEq/24 h	25–125 mmol/day

Table continued on following page

Reference Intervals for Clinical Chemistry (Urine)* Continued

	Conventional Units	SI Units
Pregnanediol		
Males	0.0–1.9 mg/24 h	0.0–6.0 μmol/day
Females		
Proliferative phase	0.0–2.6 mg/24 h	0.0–8 μmol/day
Luteal phase	2.6–10.6 mg/24 h	8–33 μmol/day
Postmenopausal	0.2–1.0 mg/24 h	0.6–3.1 μmol/day
Pregnanetriol	0.0–2.5 mg/24 h	0.0–7.4 μmol/day
Protein, total		
Qualitative	Negative	Negative
Quantitative	10–150 mg/24 h	10–150 mg/day
Protein/creatinine ratio	<0.2	<0.2
Sodium (regular diet)	60–260 mEq/24 h	60–260 mmol/day
Specific gravity		
Random specimen	1.003–1.030	1.003–1.030
24-h collection	1.015–1.025	1.015–1.025
Urate (regular diet)	250–750 mg/24 h	1.5–4.4 mmol/day
Urobilinogen	0.5–4.0 mg/24 h	0.6–6.8 μmol/day
Vanillylmandelic acid (VMA)	1.0–8.0 mg/24 h	5–40 μmol/day

Reference Intervals for Therapeutic Drug Monitoring (Serum)

	Therapeutic Range	Toxic Levels	Proprietary Names
Analgesics			
Acetaminophen	10–20 µg/mL	>250 µg/mL	Tylenol
Salicylate	100–250 µg/mL	>300 µg/mL	Disalcid
Antibiotics			
Amikacin	25–30 µg/mL	Peak: >35 µg/mL	Amikin
		Trough: >10 µg/mL	
Gentamicin	5–10 µg/mL	Peak: >10 µg/mL	Garamycin
		Trough: >2 µg/mL	
Tobramycin	5–10 µg/mL	Peak: >10 µg/mL	Nebcin
		Trough: >2 µg/mL	
Vancomycin	5–35 µg/mL	Peak: >40 µg/mL	Vancocin
		Trough: >10 µg/mL	
Anticonvulsants			
Carbamazepine	5–12 µg/mL	>15 µg/mL	Tegretol
Ethosuximide	40–100 µg/mL	>150 µg/mL	Zarontin
Phenobarbital	15–40 µg/mL	40–100 ng/mL (varies widely)	Luminal
Phenytoin	10–20 µg/mL	>20 µg/mL	Dilantin
Primidone	5–12 µg/mL	>15 µg/mL	Mysoline
Valproic acid	50–100 µg/mL	>100 µg/mL	Depakene

Table continued on following page

Reference Intervals for Therapeutic Drug Monitoring (Serum) Continued

	Therapeutic Range	Toxic Levels	Proprietary Names
Bronchodilators and Respiratory Stimulants			
Caffeine	3-15 ng/mL	>30 ng/mL	
Theophylline (aminophylline)	10-20 μg/mL	>20 μg/mL	
Cardiovascular Drugs			
Digitoxin (obtain specimen 12-24 hr after last dose)	15-25 ng/mL	>25 ng/mL	Crystodigin
Digoxin (obtain specimen more than 6 hr after last dose)	0.8-2.0 ng/mL	>2.4 ng/mL	Lanoxin
Disopyramide, serum	2-5 μg/mL	>7 μg/mL	Norpace
Flecainide	0.2-1.0 ng/mL	>1 ng/mL	Tambocor
Lidocaine, serum	1.5-5.0 μg/mL	>6 μg/mL	Xylocaine
Mexiletine	0.7-2.0 ng/mL	>2 ng/mL	Mexitil
Procainamide,	4-10 μg/mL	>12 μg/mL	Pronestyl
procainamide plus NAPA	8-30 μg/mL	>30 μg/mL	
Propranolol	50-100 ng/mL	Variable	Inderal
Quinidine	2-5 μg/mL	>6 μg/mL	Cardioquin
			Quinaglute
			Quinora
Tocainide	4-10 ng/mL	>10 ng/mL	Tonocard

Psychopharmacologic Drugs

Amitriptyline	120–150 ng/mL	>500 ng/mL	Elavil
			Triavil
Bupropion	25–100 ng/mL	Not applicable	Wellbuton
Desipramine	150–300 ng/mL	>500 ng/mL	Norpramin
Imipramine	125–250 ng/mL	>400 ng/mL	Tofranil
Lithium, serum (obtain specimen 12 hr after last dose)	0.6–1.5 mEq/L	>1.5 mEq/L	Lithobid
Nortriptyline, serum	50–150 ng/mL	>500 ng/mL	Aventyl
			Pamelor

Reference Intervals for Toxic Substances

	Conventional Units	SI Units
Arsenic, urine	<130 µ/24 h	<1.7 µmol/d
Bromides, serum, inorganic	<100 mg/dL	<10 mmol/L
Toxic symptoms	140–1000 mg/dh	14–100 mmol/L
Carboxyhemoglobin, blood:		
Urban environment	<5%	<0.05
Smokers	<12%	<0.12
Symptoms		
Headache	>15%	>0.15
Nausea and vomiting	>25%	>0.25
Potentially lethal	>50%	>0.50
Ethanol, blood	<0.05 mg/dL (<0.005%)	<1.0 mmol/L
Intoxication	>100 mg/dL (70.1%)	>22 mmol/L
Marked intoxication	300–400 mg/dL (0.3–0.4%)	65–87 mmol/L
Alcoholic stupor	400–500 mg/dL (0.4–0.5%)	87–109 mmol/L
Coma	>500 mg/dL (0.5%)	>109 mmol/L
Lead, blood		
Adults	<25 µg/dL	<1.2 µmol/L
Children	<15 µg/dL	<0.7 µmol/L
Lead, urine	<80 µg/24 h	<0.4 µmol/day
Mercury, urine	<30 µg/24 h	<150 nmol/day

Reference Intervals for Tests Performed on Cerebrospinal Fluid

	Conventional Units	SI Units
Cells	<5/mm³; all mononuclear	$<5 \times 10^6$/L, all mononuclear
Protein electrophoresis	Albumin predominant	Albumin predominant
Glucose	50–75 mg/dL	2.8–4.2 mmol/L
	(20 mg/dL less than in serum)	(1.1 mmol less than in serum)
IgG		
Children under 14	<8% of total protein	<0.08 of total protein
Adults	<14% of total protein	<0.14 of total protein
IgG index $\left(\dfrac{\text{CSF/serum IgG ratio}}{\text{CSF/serum albumin ratio}} \right)$	0.3–0.6	0.3–0.6
Oligoclonal banding on electrophoresis	Absent	Absent
Pressure, opening	70–180 mm H_2O	70–180 mm H_2O
Protein, total	15–45 mg/dL	150–450 mg/L

REFERENCE INTERVALS FOR THE INTERPRETATION OF LABORATORY TESTS

Reference Intervals for Tests of Gastrointestinal Function

Test	Conventional Units
Bentiromide	6-h urinary arylamine excretion greater than 57% excludes pancreatic insufficiency
β-Carotene, serum	60–250 ng/dL
Fecal fat estimation	
Qualitative	No fat globules seen by high-power microscope
Quantitative	<6 gm/24 h (>95% coefficient of fat absorption)
Gastric acid output	
Basal	
Males	0.0–10.5 mmol/h
Females	0.0–5.6 mmol/h
Maximum (after histamine or pentagastrin)	
Males	9.0–48.0 mmol/h
Females	6.0–31.0 mmol/h
Ratio: basal/maximum	
Males	0.0–0.31
Females	0.0–0.29
Secretin test, pancreatic fluid	
Volume	>1.8 mL/kg/h
Bicarbonate	>80 mEq/L
D-Xylose absorption test, urine	>20% of ingested dose excreted in 5 h

Rakel and Bope: Conn's Current Therapy 2001. Copyright 2001 by W.B. Saunders Company.

Test	Conventional Units	IS Units
Complement, serum		
C3	85-175 mg/dL	0.85-1.75 gm/L
C4	15-45 mg/dL	150-450 mg/L
Total hemolytic (CH_{50})	150-250 U/mL	150-250 U/mL
Immunoglobulins, serum, adult		
IgG	640-1350 mg/dL	6.4-13.5 gm/L
IgA	70-310 mg/dL	0.70-3.1 gm/L
IgM	90-350 mg/dL	0.90-3.5 gm/L
IgD	0.0-6.0 mg/dL	0.0-60 mg/L
IgE	0.0-430 ng/dL	0.0-430 µg/L

Lymphocyte Subsets, Whole Blood, Heparinized

Antigen(s) Expressed	Cell Type	Percentage	Absolute Cell Count
CD3	Total T cells	56-77%	860-1880
CD19	Total B cells	7-17%	140-370
CD3 and CD4	Helper-inducer cells	32-54%	550-1190
CD3 and CD8	Suppressor-cytotoxic cells	24-37%	430-1060
CD3 and DR	Activated T cells	5-14%	70-310
CD2	E rosette T cells	73-87%	1040-2160
CD16 and CD56	Natural killer (NK) cells	8-22%	130-500

Helper/suppressor ratio: 0.8-1.8

Rakel and Bope: Conn's Current Therapy 2001. Copyright 2001 by W.B. Saunders Company.

Reference Values for Semen Analysis

Test	Conventional Units	SI Units
Volume	2-5 mL	2-5 mL
Liquefaction	Complete in 15 min	Complete in 15 min
pH	7.2-8.0	7.2-8.0
Leukocytes	Occasional or absent	Occasional or absent
Spermatozoa		
Count	60-150×10^6 mL	60-150×10^6 mL
Motility	>80% motile	>0.80 motile
Morphology	80-90% normal forms	0.80-0.90 normal forms
Fructose	>150 mg/dL	>8.33 mmol/L

Rakel and Bope: Conn's Current Therapy 2001. Copyright 2001 by W.B. Saunders Company.

Pain, the Fifth Vital Sign

Assess for pain, now called the fifth vital sign, every time TPR and BP are taken.

Obtain the patient's description of the pain: "Pain is what the patient says it is."

Determine the characteristics of the pain.

Onset (date, sudden or gradual)

Duration (constant or intermittent)

Location (Have patient state or point to where the pain is. Mark on a body diagram)

Quality (crushing, burning, aching, throbbing, sharp, dull, etc.)

Severity/intensity (Use pain intensity scale for most objective measurement Figures A-1 and 2)

Note signs of pains

Superficial and low to moderate intensity pain

tachypnea

tachycardia

increased blood pressure

pallor

diaphoresis

increased muscle tension

pupil dilation

Severe, deep, or continuous pain

Rapid, irregular breathing

Bradycardia

Decreased blood pressure

Pallor

           Nausea and vomiting
           Weakness
      Any pain
           Bent posture
           Guarding (Holding or protecting the painful part)
           Teeth clenching
           Grimacing
           Restlessness
           Moaning
           Crying
      Chronic pain may not be accompanied by specific signs
           and symptoms

Determine if there is a pattern of the pain (relationship to time of day, activity, etc.)

Determine if there are any identifiable precipitating factors, associated symptoms, exacerbating or relieving factors).

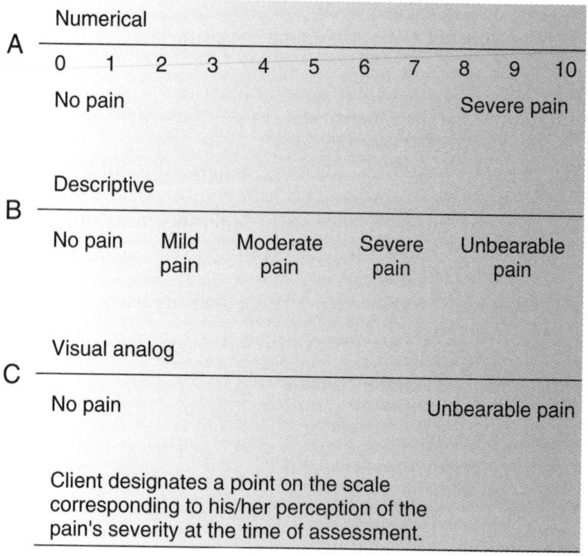

FIGURE A-1 Sample pain scales. From Potter, PA, and Perry, AG: Fundamentals of Nursing, ed. 5, St. Louis, 2001, Mosby, p. 1298.

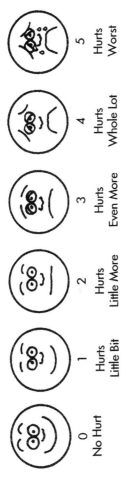

FIGURE A-2 Wong-Baker FACES Pain Rating Scale. From Wong, DL, Hockenberry-Eaton, M, Wilson, D, Winkelstein, ML, Schwartz, P: Wong's Essentials of Pediatric Nursing, ed. 6, St. Louis, 2001, p. 1301. Copyrighted by Mosby, Inc. Reprinted by permission.

Bibliography

Ablon, GR and Rosen, T. Cutaneous signs of systemic disease: a guide to gleaning diagnostic clues from the skin. Consultant, 1994 Apr; 34(4): 495–9, 503–4, 506.

Adult screening for cancer detection: thyroid examination and function: seventh in a series of articles based on chapters exerpted from the Clinician's Handbook of Clinical Preventative Services, part of the Put Prevention into Practice Program from the US Public Health Service. Nurse Pract, 1995 May; 20(5): 64, 66–7.

Andresen, G. Assessing the older patient. RN, 1998; 61(3): 46–56.

Assessing Patients. Springhouse, Pa: Springhouse, 1996.

Balakas, K and Schappe, A. Procedures in home care. Well baby assessment. Home Healthcare Nurse, 1995 Sep-Oct; 13(5): 82–84.

Barker, E and Moore, K. Neurological assessment, RN, 1992; 55(4): 28–35.

Barnes, LA. Handbook of pediatric physical diagnosis, 7th ed. Philadelphia: Lippincott, 1998.

Bateman, DE. Neurological assessment of coma. J Neurol Neurosurg Psychiatry, 2001 Sep; 71 Suppl 1: I13–I17.

Bates, B, Hoekelman, RA, et al. Guide to physical examination and history taking, 7th ed. Philadelphia: Lippincott, 1998.

Burton, M. (ed). Hall & Colman's diseases of the ear, nose and throat, 15th ed. Philadelphia: Churchill Livingstone, 2000.

Bynum, WF and Porter, R. (eds). Medicine and the five senses. New York: Cambridge University Press, 1993.

Cancer detection by physical examination: breast and pelvic organ examination. Nurs Pract, 1994 Oct; 19(10), 20–2, 24.

Caulker-Burnett, I. Primary care screening for substance abuse. Nurs Pract, 1994 Jun; 19(6): 42, 44–8.

Coulehan, JL and Block, MR. The medical interview: mastering skills for clinical practice. Philadelphia: FA Davis, 2001.

Degowin's diagnostic examination, 7th ed. New York: McGraw Hill Professional Pub, 1999.

Dermatology Nurses Association, Dermatology Nursing Essentials: A Core Curriculum. New Jersey: Anthony J Janetti Inc, 1998.

Dubowitz, V, et al. Neurological assessment of the preterm and full-term newborn infant. Clinics in Developmental Medicine Ser: No. 148 McKeith Pr GBR, 2nd ed. 2000.

Dudek, SG. Nutrition essentials for nursing practice, 4th ed. Philadelphia: Lippincott, 2001.

Edwards, SM and Murdin, L. Respiratory rate—an under-documented clinical assessment. Clin Med, 2001 Jan-Feb; 1(1): 85.

Evans-Stoner, N. Nutrition assessment: a practical approach. Nurs Clin North Am, 1997; 32(4): 637–50.

Freeborne, N. The functionally oriented assessment of the geriatric patient. Journal of the American Academy of Physician Assistants, 1994 Mar; 7(3): 158–67, 29A.

Habif, TP. Skin disease diagnosis and treatment. St. Louis: Mosby, 2001.

Jacobus, CH. Neuro assessment. Step-by-step neurological evaluation techniques for EMS providers. J Emerg Med Serv JEMS, 2000 Jan; 25(1): 56-67.

Kanski, KK. Clinical ophthalmology: a systematic approach, 4th ed. Boston: Butterworth-Heinemann, 1999.

Kelsher, KC. Primary care for women: environmental assessment of the home, community, and workplace. J Nurse Midwife, 1995 Mar-Apr; 40(2): 59–64, 88–96.

Lookingbill, DP and Marks, JG Jr. Principles of dermatology, 3rd ed. Philadelphia: WB Saunders, 2000.

McGee, SR. Evidence based physical diagnosis. Philadelphia: WB Saunders, 2001.

McGrath, A. Abdominal examination and assessment in A&E. Emerg Nurse, 1998 Jul; 6(4): 15-8.

Misulis, KE. Neurologic localization and diagnosis. Boston: Butterworth-Heinemann, 1996.

Morrissey, J. Obtaining a "reasonably accurrate" health history. Plastic Surgical Nursing, 1994 Spring; 14(1): 27–30.

Motyka, TM and Yanuck, SF. Expanding the neurological examination using functional neurologic assessment part I: methodological considerations. Int J Neurosci, 1999 Mar; 97(1–2): 61–76.

Neal, L. Is anybody home? Basic neurologic assessment of the home care client. Home Healthcare Nurse, 1997; 15(3): 156–9.

Orient, JM and Sapira, JD. Art and science of bedside diagnosis. Philadelphia: Lippincott, 2000.

Owen, A. Respiratory assessment revisited. Nursing, 1998 Apr; 28(4): 48–9.

Pressman, EK, Zeidman, SM, Summers L. Primary care for women: comprehensive assessment of the neurologic system. J Nurse Midwife, 1995 Mar-Apr; 40(2): 59–64, 163–71.

Schmitt, WH Jr and Yanuck, SF. Expanding the neurological examination using functional neurologic assessment: part II neurologic basis of applied kinesiology. Int J Neurosci, 1999 Mar; 97(1–2): 77–108.

Seidel, HM. Mosby's guide to physical examination, 4th ed. St. Louis: Mosby–Yearbook, 1998.

Seymour, CA. Clinical clerking: a short introduction to clinical skills, 2nd ed. New York: Cambridge University Press, 1994.

Shah, S. Neurological assessment. Nurs Stand, 1999 Feb 17–23; 13(22): 49–54; quiz 55–6.

Smith, DS. Field guide to bedside diagnosis. Philadelphia: Lippincott, 1999.

Swartz, MH. Textbook of physical diagnosis. History and Examination, 4th ed. Philadelphia: WB Saunders, 2001.

Talbot L and Curtis L. The challenge of assessing skin indicators in people of color. Home Healthcare Nurse, 1996; 14(3): 167–73.

Wilkins, RL, Krider, SJ, and Sheldon, RL. Clinical assessment in respiratory care, 4th ed. St. Louis: Mosby–Yearbook, 2000.

Young, RC Jr and Ford, JG. Standards for assessment of lung function and respiratory health in minority populations: some challenges linger into the new millennium. J Health Care Poor Underserved, 2001 May; 12(2): 152–61.

Young, T. Skin assessment and usual presentations. Community Nurse, 1997; 3(5): 33–36.

Index

Page numbers followed by f *refer to figures; page numbers followed by* t *refer to tables.*